Managing
LONG COVID
Syndrome

Thanthullu Vasu

tfm Publishing Limited, Castle Hill Barns, Harley, Shrewsbury, SY5 6LX, UK
Tel: +44 (0)1952 510061; Fax: +44 (0)1952 510192
E-mail: info@tfmpublishing.com; Web site: www.tfmpublishing.com

Copy-editing: Dr. Joyce Cheung BM BS, PhD, BSc (Hons)
Editing, design & typesetting: Nikki Bramhill BSc (Hons), Dip Law
Cover photo and Figure 1.1: © iStock.com
Microscopic view of the viral cell COVID-19
Credit: Julia Garan and aprott; stock illustration ID: 1214017626; 1209983819

First edition:	© 2022
Paperback	ISBN: 978-1-913755-20-1
E-book editions:	© 2022
ePub	ISBN: 978-1-913755-21-8
Mobi	ISBN: 978-1-913755-22-5
Web pdf	ISBN: 978-1-913755-23-2

Printed by Gutenberg Press Ltd., Gudja Road, Tarxien, GXQ 2902, Malta
Tel: +356 2398 2201; Fax: +356 2398 2290
E-mail: info@gutenberg.com.mt; Web site: www.gutenberg.com.mt

Contents

Section III
Guidelines and policies

Section IV
Management of long COVID syndrome

Section V
Pain management in long COVID syndrome

Section VI
Complementary therapies and pain clinic approach

Section VII
Novel pain therapies in long COVID syndrome

Section VIII
Long COVID in children

Section IX
Patient support groups for long COVID syndrome

Section X
New research interventions

Preface

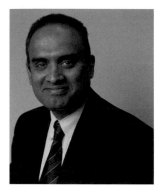

Long COVID syndrome might have been first 'discovered' by patients themselves, even before health care professionals recognised it! #LongCovid was first used by Elisa Perego from Italy in a Twitter post on 20th May 2020, describing that about 20% of patients still remained COVID-positive after 40 days, with a comment saying, 'there is a lot that we don't know about the virus'. Mentions of long COVID started appearing in newspapers, followed by use of the term by patient support groups, and it was subsequently acknowledged by the Royal College of General Practitioners in July 2020 in a BBC interview. Long COVID syndrome is one of the best examples of patient participatory medicine where patients have actively collaborated as an equal partner in managing their chronic condition and, in many cases, have led the way in lobbying and liaising with parliamentarians, health care decision-makers and financial policymakers. Unfortunately, even after a year since the term first came into use, the science underlying long COVID syndrome is still poorly understood.

I and tfm publishing are proud to be publishing one of the first books on long COVID syndrome. We have taken this opportunity to produce an easy-to-read textbook to educate and raise awareness of this new condition.

However, the disease is still relatively new, meaning scientific studies and evidence are scarce. It is commonly said that medical knowledge doubles approximately every two months; in the case of COVID-19 illness and long COVID syndrome, this will happen many times faster! To write a scientific textbook without much existing evidence is difficult and challenging. These challenges have been overcome here by applying a common-sense approach — using the best evidence available to date and extrapolating the evidence base from what is already known on other chronic conditions — and we hope that readers will be forgiving of any inaccuracies that may arise in the process. As in any field of medicine, continuous learning is always the key to the betterment of our patients.

Long COVID syndrome is a disabling and debilitating condition and can affect patients physically and psychologically, as well as their social and work life. It has a huge impact on patients' quality of life. One in ten people affected by COVID-19 illness can go on to develop long COVID syndrome. The consequence is a huge burden on the health and social care systems in the near future. Education and awareness of this condition are essential, so that health care professionals realise the need for management, managers make plans to meet service demands, policymakers construct pathways for rehabilitation and politicians make plans to meet the financial challenges of providing health care and managing the economy. Educating patients empowers them to take control of their management and helps patient support groups to lobby for their support needs in the future.

I am sure that this book will help signpost patients to appropriate services and it will help health care professionals understand the basics of the disease. It will help trainees, students and others prepare for various medical examinations. This book is written in a simple and easy-to-understand language, aiming to cater for all disciplines and specialties. If this book helps to raise awareness of long COVID syndrome and meets patients' expectations in their quest to understand the condition, then this means its goal will have been achieved.

I would like to thank Nikki Bramhill from tfm publishing who believed in my idea for this textbook and strongly supported me from the beginning, despite her very busy schedule. Her passion and dedication in publishing this book will enormously benefit many patients suffering from this condition. tfm publishing has given me endless encouragement and support. I also thank Dr. Joyce Cheung, Copy-Editor, for bearing with all my troubles and supporting me with her expertise and skills throughout this journey. Without both their help, my dream of publishing this book would not have become possible.

To all the readers, I thank you very much for reading this book. Please do not hesitate to send me your comments. All your support will be instrumental in helping to improve this book, one of the first medical texts to be published entirely on this brand new and relevant subject of long COVID syndrome. I wish you all the best for your future.

Dr. Thanthullu Vasu MBBS MD DNB FRCA FFPMRCA Dip Pain Mgt
Consultant in Pain Medicine
University Hospitals of Leicester NHS Trust, United Kingdom

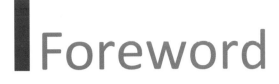Foreword

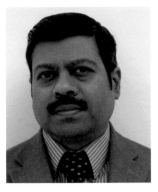

The world is yet to recover from COVID-19 but is already experiencing the deleterious effects of its long-term sequelae — post-COVID-19 syndrome or 'long COVID'. Fortunately, most people recover in weeks, but for some, symptoms are longer-lasting. Our understanding of this condition and its presentation and management is progressively increasing. While recognising the socioeconomic impact of long COVID, health care organisations throughout the world are taking initiatives to treat and support patients. For clinicians involved in providing care to people living with long-term suffering, there are currently limited resources from which to gain an overview of the condition and plan a management strategy. This concise book on the subject, *Managing long COVID syndrome*, authored by Dr. Vasu, is a timely project to meet an unmet need.

Dr. Vasu is an experienced clinician with an interest in managing long term conditions, especially pain. He has extensive clinical and academic knowledge and has published books on various medical topics, including chronic pain management. Dr. Vasu has been helping patients living with long COVID syndrome and has prepared this high-quality material based on knowledge acquired from his clinical practice and the available research evidence. The topics covered range from the cause and development of the disease to its presentation and the roles and limitations of investigations, guidelines and management. He has comprehensively included pharmacological, non-pharmacological, complementary and novel therapies to manage pain, one of the cardinal features of long COVID syndrome. The topics are presented in a succinct and simple style, with key points at the end of each chapter to help busy clinicians.

tfm publishing Ltd specialises in academic medical publishing and has previously published Dr. Vasu's work. Their partnership has produced some high-quality books widely read by multidisciplinary health care professionals. tfm publishing Ltd has presented the material in a user-friendly format. *Managing long COVID syndrome* will be a valuable addition to their range of publications. I congratulate the author and the publisher for this timely project. The book should aid clinicians in providing safe and clinically effective care and improving patients' experience.

Dr. Shyam Balasubramanian
Consultant and Associate Medical Director
UHCW NHS Trust, Coventry, United Kingdom
Honorary Associate Clinical Professor
Warwick University, United Kingdom

Abbreviations

5-HT3	5-Hydroxytryptamine-3 receptor
ACE2	Angiotensin-converting enzyme 2
ACT	Acceptance and commitment therapy
ACTH	Adrenocorticotrophic hormone
app	Application
ARDS	Acute respiratory distress syndrome
BMI	Body Mass Index
BoNT-A	Botulinum toxin type A
BoNT-B	Botulinum toxin type B
BP	Blood pressure
bpm	Beats per minute
cAMP	Cyclic adenosine monophosphate
CBT	Cognitive behavioural therapy
CBT-i	Cognitive behavioural therapy for insomnia
CCR5	C-C chemokine receptor type 5
CDC	Centers for Disease Control and Prevention
CFS	Chronic fatigue syndrome
CGRP	Calcitonin gene-related peptide
Cit-H3	Citrullated histone H3
CO_2	Carbon dioxide
COVID	Coronavirus disease
COVID-19	Coronavirus disease 2019
COX	Cyclo-oxygenase
CRP	C-reactive protein
CT	Computed tomography
CYP2D6	Cytochrome P450 enzyme
DAMP	Damage-associated molecular pattern
DN4	Douleur Neuropathique 4

DNA	Deoxyribonucleic acid
DOP	Delta opioid
ECG	Electrocardiogram
EU-OSHA	European Agency for Safety and Health at Work (European Union Information Agency for Occupational Safety and Health)
EuroQoL-5D	European Quality of Life — five dimensions
GABA	Gamma-aminobutyric acid
G-CSF	Granulocyte colony-stimulating factor
GDP	Gross domestic product
GET	Graded exercise therapy
GPCR	G-protein-coupled receptor
HCN	Hyperpolarisation-activated cyclic nucleotide gated channel
HIV	Human immunodeficiency virus
HMGB-1	High mobility group box-1
HRQL	Health-related quality of life
Hz	Hertz
IAPT	Improving Access to Psychological Therapies
ICS	Integrated care systems
IL-6	Interleukin-6
KOP	Kappa opioid
LT	Leukotriene
ME	Myalgic encephalomyelitis
MERS	Middle East respiratory syndrome
MET	Metabolic equivalent of task
MIS	Multisystem inflammatory syndrome
MOP	Mu opioid
MRI	Magnetic resonance imaging
NAPQI	N-acetyl-p-benzoquinone imine
NET	Neutrophil extracellular trap
NHS	National Health Service
NICE	National Institute for Health and Care Excellence
NIH	National Institutes of Health
NIHR	National Institute for Health Research
N/OFQ	Nociceptin/orphanin FQ

NPO	Neuropostural optimisation
NPPO-CB	Neuropsychophysical optimisation-cervicobrachial
NSAID	Non-steroidal anti-inflammatory drug
PASC	Post-acute sequelae of SARS-CoV-2 infection
PCR	Polymerase chain reaction
PEM	Post-exertional malaise
PESE	Post-exertional symptom exacerbation
PG	Prostaglandin
PGE1	Prostaglandin E1
PGE2	Prostaglandin E2
PGI2	Prostaglandin I2
PICS	Post-intensive care syndrome
PIOD	Post-infectious olfactory dysfunction
POTS	Postural orthostatic tachycardia syndrome
PPE	Personal protective equipment
PREEMPT	Phase 3 REsearch Evaluating Migraine Prophylaxis Therapy
PRINCIPLE trial	Platform Randomised Trial of Treatments in the Community for Epidemic and Pandemic Illnesses trial
PROM	Patient-reported outcome measure
PTSD	Post-traumatic stress disorder
R_0	Reproduction number (basic)
RCGP	Royal College of General Practitioners
REAC	Radioelectric asymmetric conveyer
REACT-2	REal-time Assessment of Community Transmission-2
RNA	Ribonucleic acid
SALT	Speech and language therapist
SARS	Severe acute respiratory syndrome
SARS-CoV-2	Severe acute respiratory syndrome coronavirus 2
SIGN	Scottish Intercollegiate Guidelines Network
SNAP 25	Synaptosomal-associated protein 25
SNARE	Soluble N-ethylmaleimide-sensitive factor attachment protein receptor
SNRI	Serotonin and noradrenaline reuptake inhibitor
tDCS	Transcranial direct current stimulation
TENS	Transcutaneous electrical nerve stimulation

TLR3	Toll-like receptor 3
tVNS	Transcutaneous vagal nerve stimulation
TXA2	Thromboxane A2
UK	United Kingdom
UKRI	UK Research and Innovation
UPSIT	University of Pennsylvania Smell Identification Test
USA	United States of America
WHO	World Health Organization

Section I

Long COVID syndrome

Chapter 1

Coronavirus disease

Introduction

Coronavirus disease 2019 (COVID-19) is an infectious disease caused by severe acute respiratory syndrome coronavirus 2 (SARS-CoV-2). It was first identified in Wuhan City in Hubei province, China, in December 2019, and gradually spread across the world, causing a global pandemic. Although the majority of people with COVID-19 display mild to moderate symptoms and recover, the disease can develop into serious illness, particularly in those with underlying comorbidities. Approximately 10% of people with COVID-19 will suffer persistent long-term symptoms significantly affecting their quality of life.

Aetiology

SARS-CoV-2 is a single-stranded, enveloped ribonucleic acid (RNA) virus (beta coronavirus; *Sarbecovirus* subgenus of the *Coronaviridae* family) (see ■ Figure 1.1). It was originally referred to as the 2019 novel coronavirus. It has been proposed that SARS-CoV-2 originated from animals such as bats. The virus enters human cells by binding to angiotensin-converting enzyme 2 (ACE2) receptors.

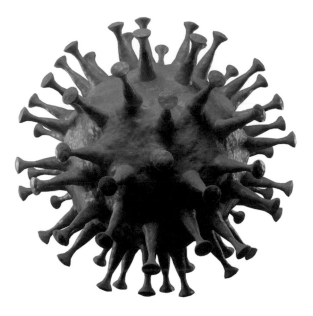

Figure 1.1. SARS-CoV-2.

SARS-CoV-2 is highly contagious. It spreads through infected saliva and respiratory secretions or respiratory droplets, as well as via aerosols. Indirect spread can also occur through contaminated surfaces, as the virus remains viable for a long time on plastic or steel surfaces. It has been found that soap deactivates the viral lipid bilayer, which stops the spread of infection.

The incubation period is estimated to be between 1 and 14 days, with a median of 5–7 days. The basic reproduction number (R_0) is estimated to be 2.2–3.3, meaning each infection can cause 2.2–3.3 further new infections in the absence of immunity. R_0 can vary significantly with new variants of the virus, depending on how contagious the infection is, and is a function of human behaviour and the biological character of the variant.

The serial interval is the time between onset of symptoms in the primary patient and that in another subsequently infected patient, and is estimated to be about 5.45 days. The secondary attack rate is the proportion of individuals exposed to the primary patient who go on to develop the disease. It is estimated to be about 7%, although it can vary depending on the virulence of the variant strain. The secondary attack rate is lower in children.

There are over 214 million confirmed cases of COVID-19 and over 4.48 million deaths caused by the disease worldwide (as of August 2021). Both the number of COVID-19 cases and the number of deaths will increase as time goes on.

Variants of SARS-CoV-2

More than 665,000 variants of SARS-CoV-2 have been sequenced to date (as of August 2021). The variants can be classified as follows:

- Variants of interest.
- Variants of concern.
- Variants of high consequence.

Further, the classification of variants can vary depending on the viral spread and country of origin. To date, four variants of concern have been designated: Alpha, Beta, Delta and Gamma.

Variants are tracked based on a naming system that uses letters of the Greek alphabet:

- Alpha: lineage B.1.1.7   variant of concern, first identified in Kent in the United Kingdom (UK) in November 2020; 50% more transmissible, causing illness with increased severity; binds more tightly to the ACE2 receptor; N501Y mutation.
- Beta: lineage B.1.351 — variant of concern, first identified in South Africa in October 2020; 50% increased transmissibility; 501.V2 mutation.

- Gamma: lineage P.1 — variant of concern, first identified in Brazil and Japan in January 2021; more transmissible and causing more severe illness.
- Delta: lineage B.1.617.2 — variant of concern, first identified in India in April 2021, was the dominant variant in the UK in the Summer of 2021; more transmissible; currently available vaccines may be effective after two doses.
- B.1.207: variant first identified in Nigeria; mutation in spike protein.
- B.1.525: variant first identified in the UK and Nigeria.
- Epsilon: lineages B.1.427 and B.1.429 — variants first identified in the United States; slightly increased transmissibility.
- Cluster 5 variant: identified in Denmark affecting mink farmers; spike protein mutation; displays resistance to antibodies; eradicated after strict quarantine.
- PANGO: lineage C.1.2 — most highly mutated variant at the time of writing (August 2021); first identified in South Africa; increased transmissibility.
- B.1.1.529: variant of concern that was dominant at the time of publication of this book, commonly called the Omicron variant; see the details overleaf.

Delta variant

The Delta variant is a variant of concern. It is more infectious, spreads faster, causes more severe illness and is at least twice more contagious than previously identified variants. It has a secondary attack rate of 11% among household contacts of PCR-positive individuals who have not travelled abroad. The Delta variant has a higher risk of hospitalisation among infected people. However, there is evidence that vaccination reduces the risk of infection, as well as preventing hospitalisation and death. Further, fully vaccinated individuals who are infected with the Delta variant have been found to exhibit a shorter period of infection.

Omicron variant (PANGO lineage B.1.1.529)

It was just before the publication of this book (December 2021), when Omicron was becoming the dominant variant of concern in many parts of the world. It was first reported in South Africa on 24th November 2021. It is a highly divergent variant with a high number of mutations, including 26-32 mutations in the spike protein of the virus. It is more contagious and is believed to spread 70 times faster in the airways of infected patients. In December 2021, it was identified in at least 110 countries and was noted to have a doubling time of only 2-3 days. Early data showed a reduced risk of hospitalisation and intensive care admissions, but more details are yet to be ascertained at the time of publication of this book.

Key Points

- COVID-19 is caused by SARS-CoV-2, previously referred to as the 2019 novel coronavirus.
- The median incubation period is 5–7 days.
- The basic reproduction number (R_0) is 2.2–3.3 but can vary significantly.
- Many thousands of mutant variants have been identified, of which the Omicron variant is predominant in many countries (at the time of writing).
- Approximately 10% of people with COVID-19 suffer persistent long-term symptoms.

References

1. World Health Organization. Coronavirus. Available from: https://www.who.int/health-topics/coronavirus#tab=tab_1.

2. Center for Systems Science and Engineering (CSSE) at John Hopkins University. COVID-19 Dashboard. Available from: https://gisanddata.maps.arcgis.com/apps/opsdashboard/index.html#/bda7594740fd40299423467b48e9ecf6.

3. Centers for Disease Control and Prevention (updated 31st August 2021). SARS-CoV-2 variant classifications and definitions. Available from: https://www.cdc.gov/coronavirus/2019-ncov/cases-updates/variant-surveillance/variant-info.html.

4. BMJ Best Practice. Coronavirus disease 2019 (COVID-19). Available from: https://bestpractice.bmj.com/topics/en-gb/3000201/aetiology.

5. Scheepers C, Everatt J, Amoako DG, *et al.* The continuous evolution of SARS-CoV-2 in South Africa: a new lineage with rapid accumulation of mutations of concern and global detection. doi: https://doi.org/10/1101/2021.08.20.21262342. Available from: https://www.medrxiv.org/content/10.1101/2021.08.20.21262342v2.

6. World Health Organization (23rd December 2021). Enhancing readiness for Omicron (B.1.1.529): Technical brief and priority actions for member states. Available from: https://www.who.int/publications/m/item/enhancing-readiness-for-omicron-(b.1.1.529)-technical-brief-and-priority-actions-for-member-states.

Chapter 2

What is long COVID syndrome?

Introduction

COVID-19 symptoms can persist for weeks or months post-illness, even after the infection itself has subsided. This is generally referred to as post-COVID-19, or long coronavirus disease (COVID), syndrome or post-acute sequelae of COVID-19 (PASC). However, there is a difference in terminology, as explained below. In general, if symptoms have persisted for 4 weeks post-infection, the condition is defined as long COVID syndrome.

Presentation of long COVID syndrome

Long COVID syndrome can affect between 1 in 5 and 1 in 10 people infected with SARS-CoV-2. The majority of people with long COVID syndrome have been previously hospitalised with severe illness, especially those with symptoms of fatigue and shortness of breath. However, long COVID syndrome can also occur in those who have mild infection not requiring hospitalisation.

The World Health Organization (WHO), in October 2020, commented that a significant number of people with COVID-19 will develop serious long-term effects, including predominantly symptoms of fatigue, headaches, exhaustion, mood swings and chronic pain. 'Brain fog', anxiety and stress are also commonly seen in patients who suffer from long COVID syndrome.

Health impact of long COVID syndrome

It has been said that the chronic needs of these 'long-haulers' have been overlooked. This has even been called a 'third-wave problem' (after the first two waves of the COVID pandemic, each causing a health care crisis). COVID-19 can cause irreversible pulmonary scarring and respiratory impairment. Cognitive dysfunction has been clearly documented, even in those with mild symptoms, with one-third of affected COVID-19 patients reported to develop neurological symptoms. A study from the UK showed that 20% of COVID-19 patients have paranoid hallucinations, confusion and agitation, and 42% suffer from delirium.

The National Institute for Health Research (NIHR) published two themed reviews in October 2020 and March 2021, respectively, aimed at providing a better understanding of long COVID syndrome. Seventy-one percent of surveyed patients with long COVID syndrome reported that the condition affected their family life; 39% said that it impacted their ability to care for their dependants; 80% described the condition impacted their ability to work, while 36% said that it affected their finances. The reviews concluded that long COVID syndrome is highly debilitating, with some people needing help with personal care, even months after the initial infection.

Definition of long COVID syndrome

The National Institute for Health and Care Excellence (NICE) has published guidelines that define the clinical manifestations of COVID-19 illness at different times into four categories (see ■ Figure 2.1):

- Acute COVID-19: signs and symptoms that last for up to 4 weeks post-infection.
- Ongoing symptomatic COVID-19: symptoms that persist for 4–12 weeks post-infection.
- Post-COVID-19 syndrome: signs and symptoms that develop either during an infection or post-infection consistent with COVID-19, and that continue for >12 weeks and are not explained by an alternative diagnosis.

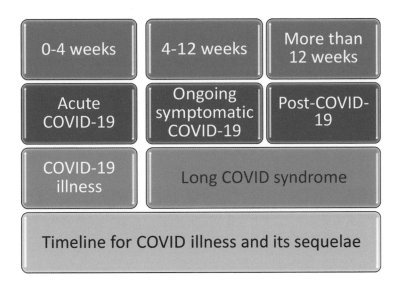

Figure 2.1. Time course for COVID-19.

- Long COVID syndrome: includes both ongoing symptomatic COVID-19 and post-COVID-19 syndrome.

Despite the above categorisation of COVID-19 illness, it remains very difficult to differentiate among the complex presentations of its sequelae post-acute illness. In clinical practice, long COVID syndrome is a commonly used term for persistent COVID-19-related clinical features.

Recognising and managing long COVID syndrome

According to the ME Association, data collected via the COVID-19 tracker app show that >12% of patients with COVID-19 report having symptoms of the illness for longer than 30 days, with debilitating fatigue being the predominant symptom.

At present, there is no tool available that can predict the duration of these symptoms. There is scientific evidence in support of a multimodal biopsychosocial model of symptom management. Supported self-management is the key to recovery in the majority of patients with long COVID syndrome, although some may require a specialist approach, as will be discussed in later chapters.

Key Points

- Long COVID syndrome affects about 1 in 10 patients.
- NICE distinguishes four different types of clinical presentations of the sequelae of COVID-19 post-acute illness.
- Symptoms lasting for >4 weeks are collectively referred to as long COVID syndrome.
- If symptoms or signs last for >12 weeks, the condition is known as post-COVID-19 syndrome.
- Long COVID syndrome will represent a major problem impacting health care delivery in the future.

References

1. National Institute for Health Research (2021). Themed review: Living with Covid19 — second review. Available from: https://evidence.nihr.ac.uk/themedreview/living-with-covid19-second-review/.
2. National Institute for Health Research (2020). Themed review: Living with Covid19 — first review. Available from: https://evidence.nihr.ac.uk/themedreview/living-with-covid19/.

3.   United Nations (2020). Long-term symptoms of COVID-19 'really concerning', says WHO chief. Available from: https://news.un.org/en/story/2020/10/1076562.

4.   Baker HA, Safavynia SA, Evered LA. The 'third wave': impending cognitive and functional decline in COVID-19 survivors. *Br J Anaesth* 2021; 126: 44–7.

5.   Mao L, Jin H, Wang M, *et al*. Neurologic manifestations of hospitalized patients with Coronavirus disease 2019 in Wuhan, China. *JAMA Neurol* 2020; 77: 683–90.

6.   Helms J, Kremer S, Merdji H, *et al*. Neurologic features in severe SARS-CoV-2 infection. *N Engl J Med* 2020; 382: 2268–70.

7.   McLoughlin BC, Miles A, Webb TE, et al. Functional and cognitive outcomes after COVID-19 delirium. *Eur Geriatr Med* 2020; 11: 857–62.

8.   National Institute for Health and Care Excellence (2020). COVID-19 rapid guideline: managing the long-term effects of COVID-19. NICE guideline [NG188]. Available from: https://www.nice.org.uk/guidance/ng188.

9.   Shepherd C (2020). Post COVID-19 fatigue, post/long COVID-19 syndromes and post-COVID ME/CFS. Available from: https://meassociation.org.uk/wp-content/uploads/MEA-Covid-19-MECFS-Post-Covid-Fatigue-Syndromes-and-Management-November-2020.pdf.

Chapter 3

Epidemiology of long COVID syndrome

Introduction

The COVID-19 pandemic has led to a major global health care crisis. As of 27th August 2021, over 214 million cases of COVID-19 have been confirmed worldwide, with more than 4.48 million deaths. Long COVID syndrome can markedly affect quality of life and can become a significant burden to society. In addition to its physical and psychological implications, long COVID syndrome also bears social consequences as it affects both patients and their families. A study showed that 17.8% of individuals who were working prior to being infected with SARS-CoV-2 were no longer in active employment, while 19.3% had a change in their work status due to the negative impact of the infection on their health.

Prevalence in the United Kingdom

It is estimated that around 10% of people with COVID-19 suffer from long COVID syndrome.

In the UK, more than 1 million people are estimated to suffer from long COVID symptoms (as of 2nd May 2021), accounting for 1.6% of the UK population. It is highly likely that there could be many more affected patients who have not reported long COVID symptoms. Two-thirds of those with long

COVID syndrome have reported a negative impact of the condition on their day-to-day activities. Of the 1 million affected, more than 37.6% had long COVID symptoms persisting for more than 1 year after the initial COVID-19 infection!

Data from the above survey showed that the most commonly reported symptoms were fatigue (54.7%), followed by shortness of breath (40.5%), muscle pain (31.3%) and concentration difficulties (28.5%).

In the recent REal-time Assessment of Community Transmission-2 (REACT-2) study, researchers from the Imperial College London conducted a survey of 508,707 patients who were asked about the presence of 29 different COVID-related symptoms. The findings confirmed an incidence of 37.7% of severe, persistent symptoms 12 weeks after SARS-CoV-2 infection, giving a weighted prevalence of long COVID syndrome of 5.75% in the general population. This study estimated that more than 2 million people in England have been affected by long COVID syndrome (as of 28th June 2021), with almost one-third (30.5%) reporting severe symptoms.

Prevalence after hospital discharge in the UK

Another UK study investigating organ-specific dysfunction in 47,780 patients with COVID-19 illness who were discharged from hospital found significantly higher rates of respiratory disease, diabetes and cardiovascular disease in these patients, with 770, 127 and 126 diagnoses per 1000 person-years, respectively. These results showed that patients have increased rates of multiorgan dysfunction when discharged from hospital after COVID-19 illness, compared with the expected risk in the general population.

The same study found almost a third of these patients were readmitted to hospital, as well as a greater risk of death in these patients (7.7 times greater than in matched controls).

Prevalence in other countries

- A Swedish study of young, healthy health care workers found that 26% of COVID-19-positive participants reported persistent moderate to severe symptoms after 2 months. The most common symptoms were anosmia, fatigue, ageusia and shortness of breath. Of these participants, 8% reported that their long-term symptoms disrupted their work life from moderate to severe levels; 15% of the participants reported that their symptoms impacted their social life, and 11% reported disability using the Sheehan Disability Scale.
- An observational study conducted in the United States reported an incidence of 32.6% of persistent symptoms in patients with COVID-19, with 15.1% needing hospital readmission. Dyspnoea was the most common clinical feature in these patients.
- An outpatient Italian clinic described symptom persistence in 87.4% of patients at 60 days post-COVID-19 illness, with fatigue, shortness of breath and joint and chest pain as commonly reported symptoms. Further, the EuroQoL-5D scale showed a decline in the quality of life in 44.1% of patients who had persistent symptoms at 60 days post-COVID-19 illness.
- A French study showed an incidence of long COVID syndrome in two-thirds of patients at 60 days post-diagnosis of COVID-19.
- A prospective cohort study carried out in Wuhan, China, reported that 76% of patients who had COVID-19 had at least one symptom of long COVID syndrome at 6 months from symptom onset. Fatigue and muscle weakness were the most commonly reported symptoms (63%), followed by sleep difficulties (26%).
- A recent meta-analysis of available literature in May 2021 from various countries described an estimated prevalence of 10–35% of post-COVID syndrome — a figure likely significantly higher in patients who were hospitalised due to COVID-19 illness, compared to those who were managed at home.
- A survey conducted by the US Department of Veterans Affairs based on the national health care database showed a higher risk of death, as well as increased health resource utilisation, beyond the first 30 days of illness among individuals with COVID-19.

Demographics

A higher prevalence of long COVID syndrome has been reported in the following groups:

- Females.
- People aged 35–69 years.
- People living in deprived areas.
- People working in health and social care sectors.
- People with an activity-limiting health condition or disability.

Predictors and risk factors

Risk factors associated with long COVID syndrome include increasing age, high body mass index and female sex. In patients with more than five COVID-related symptoms in the first week of illness, their risk of developing long COVID syndrome is increased more than threefold (odds ratio of 3.53).

Key Points

- It is estimated that up to 10% of patients with COVID-19 suffer from long COVID syndrome.
- More than 1.6% of the UK population are affected by long COVID syndrome.
- Long COVID syndrome has a negative impact on the quality of life in two-thirds of affected patients.

References

1. World Health Organization. Coronavirus disease (COVID-19). Available from: https://www.who.int/health-topics/coronavirus#tab=tab_1.

2. Office for National Statistics (2021). Prevalence of ongoing symptoms following coronavirus (COVID-19) infection in the UK: 4 June 2021. Available from: https://www.ons.gov.uk/peoplepopulationand community/healthandsocialcare/conditionsanddiseases/bulletins/prevalenceofongoingsymptoms followingcoronaviruscovid19infectionintheuk/4June2021.

3. BMJ Opinion (2021). Long covid — looking across data, diseases, and disciplines. Available from: https://blogs.bmj.com/bmj/2021/03/31/long-covid-looking-across-data-diseases-and-disciplines/.

4. Alford J (2021). Over 2 million adults in England may have had long COVID — Imperial REACT. Available from: https://www.imperial.ac.uk/news/224853/over-million-adults-england-have-long/.

5. Whitaker M, Elliott J, Chadeau-Hyam M, *et al* (2021). Persistent symptoms following SARS-CoV-2 infection in a random community sample of 508,707 people. Available from: https://spiral.imperial.ac.uk/handle/10044/1/89844.

6. Ayoubkhani D, Khunti K, Nafilyan V, *et al.* Post-covid syndrome in individuals admitted to hospital with covid-19: retrospective cohort study. *BMJ* 2021; 372: n693.

7. Sudre CH, Murray B, Varsavsky T, *et al.* Attributes and predictors of long COVID. *Nat Med* 2021; 27: 626–31.

8. Nalbandian A, Sehgal K, Gupta A, *et al.* Post-acute COVID-19 syndrome. *Nat Med* 2021; 27: 601–15.

9. The Health Foundation (2021). What might long COVID mean for the nation's health? Available from: https://www.health.org.uk/news-and-comment/blogs/what-might-long-covid-mean-for-the-nations-health.

10. Haverall S, Rosell A, Phillipson M. Symptoms and functional impairment assessed 8 months after mild COVID-19 among health care workers. *JAMA* 2020; 325: 2015–6.

11. Al-Aly Z, Xie Y, Bowe B. High dimensional characterization of post-acute sequelae of COVID-19. *Nature* 2021; 594: 259–64.

12. Pavli A, Theodoridou M, Maltezou HC. Post-COVID syndrome: incidence, clinical spectrum, and challenges for primary healthcare professionals. *Arch Med Res* 2021; 52: 575–81.

Chapter 4

Aetiopathogenesis of long COVID syndrome

Introduction

Various theories have been proposed for the aetiopathogenesis of long COVID syndrome (see ■ Figure 4.1). In acute COVID illness, SARS-CoV-2 causes damage to the immune and microvascular systems, as well as to the endothelium. It also affects the angiotensin-converting enzyme 2 (ACE2) pathway, resulting in a hyperinflammatory state, cytokine storm, hypercoagulability and thrombosis. Below are some of the various theories explaining the aetiopathogenesis of long COVID syndrome.

Long-term immunological changes

In response to acute SARS-CoV-2 infection, it is possible that immunological changes continue to persist for a long time, causing damage to various organs, including the lungs and the heart. Evidence of pulmonary fibrosis, downregulation of ACE2 receptors and fibrofatty changes in the myocardium as a result of SARS-CoV-2 infection could support this theory to explain the persistence of symptoms that lead to long COVID syndrome.

Similarly to SARS-CoV-2 infection, autoimmune or inflammatory mechanisms have also been proposed to underlie other viral infections such as those caused by the Chikungunya virus, Ebola virus and Epstein-Barr virus.

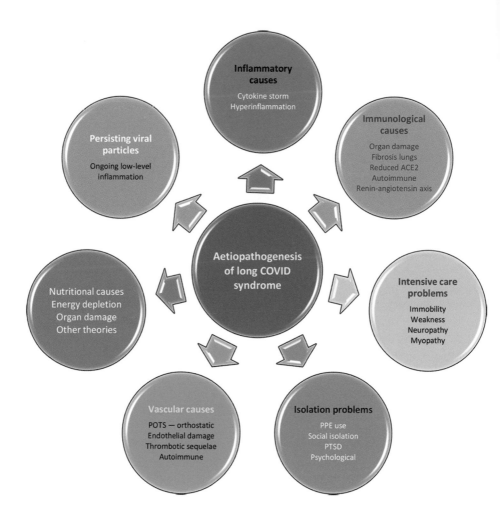

Figure 4.1. Aetiopathogenesis of long COVID syndrome. ACE2 = angiotensin-converting enzyme 2; POTS = postural orthostatic tachycardia syndrome; PTSD = post-traumatic stress disorder; PPE = personal protective equipment.

Post-intensive care syndrome

It is well recognised that patients with long stays in the intensive care unit due to various medical conditions can suffer from post-critical care syndrome involving myopathy and neuropathy. This is especially common after long-term ventilation and use of muscle relaxants. It has been proposed that COVID illness is also associated with similar muscular weakness, especially with a prolonged acute stage accompanied by a cytokine storm and long intensive care stay. This pathophysiological theory could be supported by the phylogenetic similarities between SARS-CoV-2 and other coronaviruses such as the severe acute respiratory syndrome (SARS) coronavirus and Middle East respiratory syndrome (MERS) coronavirus. Further, immobility, use of various drugs, metabolic changes and microvascular ischaemia are also some of the factors contributing to post-intensive care syndrome.

Persistent inflammation

Prolonged inflammation plays a key role in causing the majority of post-COVID symptoms. Long-term neurological symptoms result from the hyperinflammatory acute phase.

Some research groups have postulated that ongoing low-level inflammation in the brain is responsible for many signs and symptoms of long COVID syndrome, including brain fog. High cytokine levels during acute illness have been found to be associated with migraine-like headaches. Neuroinflammation and microvascular changes in the brain are thought to be the cause of malaise and fatigue that occur in long COVID syndrome.

Neuroinflammation leading to decreased gamma-aminobutyric acid (GABA) levels, caused by reduced density of GABA receptors, could possibly explain the fatigue and cognitive changes observed in long COVID syndrome. There is evidence for raised protein markers of nerve dysfunction in these patients.

Vascular and autonomic nervous systems

Decreased cerebral blood flow and changes in the autonomic nervous system have been proposed to be responsible for the persistent signs and symptoms of long COVID syndrome. A proportion of patients with long COVID syndrome suffer from postural hypotension and tachycardia syndrome, especially in the first 3–6 months after an acute infection. Thrombotic complications requiring anticoagulation can also be prolonged in some patients.

Pulmonary fibrosis

Acute COVID-19 illness causes pulmonary fibrosis, which could explain the respiratory sequelae in long COVID syndrome; this is commonly seen in severe acute respiratory distress syndrome (ARDS) associated with COVID-19. The prevalence of dyspnoea lasting 60–100 days post-COVID-19 illness has been estimated to be 42–66%. Endothelial damage in acute illness has been found to be associated with extravasation of protein-rich fluid into the alveolar space, causing significant lung damage. There is also an increased incidence of pulmonary fibrosis with the occurrence of a cytokine storm.

Organ damage

Chronic organ inflammation can cause persistence of symptoms in the convalescent phase. If these symptoms are not managed appropriately in a timely manner, this could lead to deconditioning and chronic illness. The severity of the acute illness depends on the extent of organ damage as a result of inflammation.

Psychosocial factors

COVID-19 can cause significant post-traumatic stress and depression. Not only does the associated organ damage cause psychological issues, but also the use of personal protective equipment (PPE), isolation and social impact can all contribute to the multifactorial pathophysiology of long COVID syndrome. Social factors, including job loss, financial problems, loss of a family member or close friend and changes in family dynamics, can lead to deconditioning and prolongation of the illness. As in any chronic condition, the use of a biopsychosocial model to manage long COVID syndrome can have positive outcomes.

Dysregulation of the renin-angiotensin-aldosterone system

Since SARS-CoV-2 acts on ACE2 receptors, it has been proposed that receptor changes could lead to dysregulation of the renin-angiotensin-aldosterone system. It is possible this can persist for prolonged periods in some patients.

Energy substrate depletion

Energy depletion due to substrate deficiency has been proposed as another mechanism underlying the development of long COVID syndrome, although direct evidence is yet to be obtained. This could explain the manifestation of fatigue that is commonly seen in patients with long COVID syndrome.

Cellular changes

It is possible that SARS-CoV-2 itself directly causes changes at a cellular level that could result in fatigue.

Key Points

- A number of theories based on multisystem involvement have been proposed to explain the persistence of signs and symptoms in long COVID syndrome.
- Immune dysregulation and persistent inflammatory changes could underlie the persistent nature of long COVID manifestations.
- There are similarities between long COVID patients and patients on long-term ventilation in terms of the development of post-critical care syndrome, although more organs/systems can be involved and the condition can last longer in long COVID syndrome.
- Since SARS-CoV-2 binds to ACE2 receptors, dysregulation of the renin-angiotensin-aldosterone system can cause long-term symptoms.
- As long COVID syndrome is highly debilitating, patients are best managed by adopting a biopsychosocial approach.

References

1. Nalbandian A, Sehgal K, Gupta A, et al. Post-acute COVID-19 syndrome. Nat Med 2021; 27: 601–15.

2. Komaroff AL (2021). The tragedy of long COVID. Harvard Health Publishing. Available from: https://www.health.harvard.edu/blog/the-tragedy-of-the-post-covid-long-haulers-202010152479.

3. Raveendran AV, Jayadevan R, Sashidharan S. Long COVID: an overview. Diabetes Metab Syndr 2021; 15: 869–75.

4. Maltezou HC, Pavli A, Tsakris A. Post-COVID syndrome: an insight on its pathogenesis. Vaccines (Basel) 2021; 9: 497.

Chapter 5

Prolonged clinical manifestations of post-acute COVID-19

Introduction

Many people improve clinically a few days or weeks following an acute infection with SARS-CoV-2. Studies have shown that the majority recover fully within 12 weeks. However, a proportion of COVID-19 patients will suffer persistent symptoms of long COVID syndrome with multisystemic involvement. This chapter gives an introduction to the multisystemic manifestations of long COVID syndrome (these will be individually dealt with in detail in later chapters).

Signs and symptoms of long COVID syndrome

Various studies have found no correlation between the initial acute infection and its severity and the risk of long-term symptoms. Even non-hospitalised patients with mild symptoms can suffer from long COVID syndrome.

Common signs and symptoms that persist long after acute COVID-19 are oulined in ■ Table 5.1 overleaf.

Table 5.1. Common signs and symptoms that persist long after acute COVID-19.

Respiratory:
- Shortness of breath
- Persistent cough

Cardiovascular:
- Chest pain
- Chest tightness
- Palpitations
- Dizziness and fainting
- Postural hypotension
- Posture-related tachycardia
- Tachycardia

Neurological:
- 'Brain fog'
- Difficulty to concentrate
- Cognitive impairment
- Memory problems
- Generalised weakness
- Headache
- Delirium

Ear, nose and throat:
- Reduced or loss of taste sensation, metallic taste, altered taste sensation
- Reduced or loss of smell sensation
- Sore throat
- Tinnitus and vertigo
- Dizziness
- Earache
- Difficulty swallowing

Dermatological:
- Skin rashes

Peripheral neuropathy:
- Pins and needles, tingling
- Other forms of paraesthesiae

Pain:
- Chronic pain
- Musculoskeletal pain
- Widespread dysaesthesia
- Multiple joint pain

Psychiatric/psychological:
- Low mood, frustration, depression, changes in mood
- Anxiety
- Panic attacks
- Post-traumatic stress disorder (PTSD)

Sleep problems:
- Insomnia
- Poor sleep quality, feeling tired on waking
- Excessive sleep and tiredness
- Interrupted sleep

Gastrointestinal:
- Nausea and vomiting
- Abdominal pain
- Diarrhoea
- Reduced appetite
- Anorexia

Other:
- Fatigue
- Persistent low-grade fever
- Recurrent fever

Brain fog and fatigue are the commonest symptoms.

These signs and symptoms can overlap and even fluctuate. Studies have described 205 different long-term symptoms in ten different organ systems, with 66 symptoms detected over 7 months. Symptoms have also been reported to worsen after physical or mental activities.

The REACT-2 study on long COVID symptoms

The recent REal-time Assessment of Community Transmission 2 (REACT-2) study, conducted by Imperial College London, has reported an incidence of 6% of significant systemic problems in patients who had COVID-19, after 12 weeks or more following acute illness.

According to the study, it is estimated that there are more than 2 million people suffering from long COVID syndrome in England (as of June 2021). The REACT-2 study identified two patient groups:

- A smaller group of patients with severe respiratory symptoms (shortness of breath, chest tightness, chest pain).
- A larger group of patients with tiredness, muscle aches and sleep problems.

Other studies

A recent study on an international cohort of long COVID patients examined the symptom profile over 7 months in 3762 patients. Findings showed that 96% of patients had symptoms beyond 90 days, with an estimated total of 205 symptoms in ten organ systems, and sufferers had an average of 14.5 symptoms affecting an average of nine organ systems. These results showed that long COVID syndrome has a multisystemic impact, leading to an overlap of symptoms that are difficult to manage without a multidisciplinary approach. The study also found the commonest symptoms at 6 months were fatigue (77%), post-exertional malaise (72%) and cognitive dysfunction (55%).

A study using data from the national health care database of the US Department of Veterans Affairs identified persistent symptoms in patients many months post-acute COVID-19, including sequelae affecting the respiratory and nervous systems, neurocognitive disorders, mental health disorders, metabolic disorders, cardiovascular disorders, gastrointestinal disorders, malaise, fatigue, musculoskeletal pain and anaemia.

Multisystem inflammatory syndrome (MIS) following COVID-19 illness has also been reported to affect multiple body systems, including the heart, lungs, kidneys, skin and brain. It is possible that autoimmune changes can affect multiple organs in this way.

Postural orthostatic tachycardia syndrome

Patients with COVID-19 can develop symptoms of light-headedness, palpitations and fainting post-acute illness that persist for prolonged periods. Standing upright can cause dizziness in these patients. These symptoms, as well as orthostatic hypotension, are caused by an impaired response of the autonomic nervous system to changes in posture.

Postural orthostatic tachycardia syndrome (POTS) is diagnosed by the active stand test whereby blood pressure and heart rate are measured after 5 minutes of lying supine and then after 3 minutes of standing. Orthostatic hypotension is present if there is a drop in systolic blood pressure (BP) of >20mmHg and in diastolic BP of >10mmHg. POTS is also associated with an increase in heart rate of >30 beats per minute when standing.

Psychological impact

Anxiety and depression are common symptoms reported in patients with long COVID syndrome. Mental health problems are worse in patients who have had prolonged stays in intensive care during the acute illness. Tiredness, joint pain and generalised pain impact on quality of life and can even lead to identity loss as patients lose their role in society.

Patients have reported suffering from PTSD after severe infections, especially those who were hospitalised during their COVID-19 illness. The use of personal protective equipment (PPE), isolation from family and multiple invasive clinical interventions, as well as fear of the unknown, can all lead to PTSD in these patients.

Social impact

Job loss, as well as loss of income, can lead to significant family and social problems. People on furlough (financial support towards wages given to full-time workers in some developed countries, including the UK, to avoid job losses during lockdowns) who had COVID-19 have also found their lives affected at a later stage when the furlough scheme ended.

Key Points

- Persistent symptoms after acute COVID-19 can affect multiple body systems, leading to various clinical presentations.
- Two separate patient groups are recognised: those with severe respiratory symptoms and those with fatigue, pain and sleep problems.
- Postural hypotension is a recognised symptom in long COVID syndrome.
- The multisystemic manifestations of long COVID syndrome impact patients' psychological and social well-being.

References

1.   NHS (2021). Long-term effects of coronavirus (long COVID). Available from: https://www.nhs.uk/conditions/coronavirus-covid-19/long-term-effects-of-coronavirus-long-covid/.

2.   Imperial College London (2021). Over 2 million adults in England may have had long COVID — Imperial REACT. Available from: https://www.imperial.ac.uk/news/224853/over-million-adults-england-have-long/.

3.   Centers for Disease Control and Prevention (2021). Post-COVID conditions. Available from: https://www.cdc.gov/coronavirus/2019-ncov/long-term-effects.html.

4.   Davis HE, Assaf GS, McCorkell L, *et al.* Characterizing long COVID in an international cohort: 7 months of symptoms and their impact. *EClinicalMedicine* 2021; 38: 101019.

5.   Dani M, Dirksen A, Taraborrelli P, *et al.* Autonomic dysfunction in 'long COVID': rationale, physiology and management strategies. *Clin Med J* 2021; 21: e63–7.

6.   Al-Aly Z, Xie Y, Bowe B. High-dimensional characterization of post-acute sequelae of COVID-19. *Nature* 2021; 594: 259–64.

Chapter 6

Problems after intensive care stay in COVID-19 patients

Introduction

The COVID-19 pandemic has taught us many lessons in health care resource utilisation and allocation. Possibly one of the most important lessons is in the appropriate management of intensive care resources, including beds and oxygen supply. In all health care institutions across the world, the existing number of intensive care beds in the pre-pandemic era has proven scarce and inadequate to meet the surging demands in bed capacity during the pandemic. New Nightingale hospitals (special temporary hospitals reserved for COVID-19 patients in the UK) were thus set up as an urgent measure. However, intensive care stay has resulted in its own set of long-term problems in patients who were admitted into intensive care for COVID-19 and survived.

Post-intensive care syndrome: long-term sequelae following intensive care stay

Post-intensive care syndrome (PICS) is known to occur in many patients following their stay in intensive care units, with the development of long-term physical symptoms of weakness, breathlessness and tiredness. PICS also encompasses mental health and cognitive impairment, including depression, anxiety and memory and concentration problems (see ■ Figure 6.1). A previous 5-year longitudinal study on intensive care patients with acute respiratory distress syndrome (ARDS) showed that psychiatric symptoms,

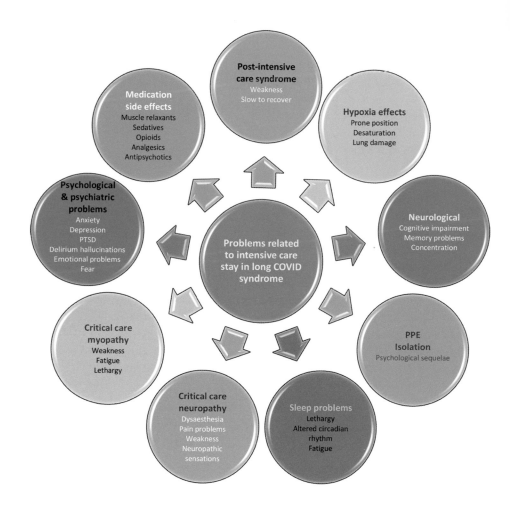

Figure 6.1. Long-term sequelae following intensive care stay in COVID-19 patients.

including symptoms of anxiety, depression and post-traumatic stress disorder (PTSD), can persist in the long term.

Problems specific to COVID-19 illness

COVID-19 has worsened the incidence of PICS, mainly due to two factors:

- Fear of this new fatal disease is likely to result in significant catastrophising.
- Use of personal protective equipment (PPE) and severe restrictions imposed on direct interactions with family/friends (as part of infection control measures) can lead to significant emotional difficulties.

Sleep disturbances and delirium

The intensive care environment is one of the busiest and noisiest in the hospital, and consequently, patients staying in intensive care experience disruption in their circadian rhythm. Delirium can be due to either the systemic illness itself (such as fever, sepsis, inflammation, etc.) or side effects of medications used (such as sedatives, analgesics, muscle relaxants, anti-histaminergics, etc.). Patients are known to have vivid hallucinations and dreams that could lead to the development of PTSD. The use of ventilatory support and fear of the unknown can significantly impact patients' psychological status.

Cognitive impairment

It is well known that patients who had prolonged intensive care stay suffer from long-term cognitive impairment, and this was evident even before the COVID-19 pandemic. A 2013 study showed that 74% of patients, who were admitted for various medical causes, developed delirium during their intensive care stay. In this study, even at 1 year post-intensive care stay, 34% of older, and 24% of younger, patients had persistent cognitive deficits, with similar cognition scores to patients with moderate traumatic brain injury and those with mild Alzheimer's disease, respectively. Cognitive impairment in

COVID-19 patients post-intensive care stay manifests as deficits in memory, attention and executive function.

Lessons learnt from past experience: SARS outbreak

The long-term psychological and social sequelae of the SARS outbreak in 2003 has been studied in detail. Studies reported that 33% of SARS patients suffered from significant mental health problems even at 1 year post-illness. Factors described by patients that contributed to their mental stress include social stigma, loss of anonymity through social media and death of close family members or colleagues, as well as an inability to attend their funeral. The mental health impact as a consequence of the COVID-19 pandemic is likely to be worse, given that many affected patients have lost their loved ones and had no opportunity to deal appropriately with their loss due to quarantine and isolation rules.

Critical care neuropathy

Neuropathy is a well-known condition affecting patients with a long intensive care stay. The incidence of neuropathy is increased by the use of muscle relaxants to facilitate ventilatory support.

Critical care myopathy

Prolonged bed rest and immobility, as is the case in intensive care, can lead to disuse atrophy. Many patients experience weakness following their discharge from intensive care after a long stay. The main complaint is that of fatigue, even after minimal effort, which can limit patients' daily activities and affect their quality of life and recovery. Critical care myopathy has been shown to be worse in COVID-19 patients than in any other group of intensive care patients.

Prone positioning in intensive care to improve oxygenation

Prone positioning of intensive care patients is commonly adopted in severe or persistent hypoxaemia. However, proning can result in prolonged muscle weakness and widespread joint pain. Position-associated skin damage or bed sores can also cause pain exacerbation, along with delayed recovery. Inappropriate support during proning leads to peripheral neuropathies that can persist even after patient recovery.

Chronic pain after COVID-19-related intensive care admission

Joint pain, generalised pain, myalgia and chest pain are all typical features of long COVID syndrome. A recent analysis of intensive care in the UK found that two-thirds of patients with COVID-19 who were admitted into intensive care experienced new ongoing pain following their discharge from the intensive care unit.

Admission into intensive care not only carries high mortality rates during patients' stay in the unit, but also increases the risk of post-discharge mortality. A French cross-sectional study using hospital discharge data reported a mortality rate of 72.1% at 6 months post-hospital discharge among patients aged over 80 years who received ventilatory support for COVID-19 during their intensive care stay.

Key Points

- PICS is a condition known to occur frequently among ARDS and intensive care patients.
- COVID-19 presents difficult challenges: fear of the unknown and problems secondary to the use of PPE/social isolation.
- Cognitive disturbances occur, even many months after discharge from intensive care.
- Critical care myopathy and neuropathy are significant long-term problems in patients with prolonged intensive care stay.
- Chronic pain is a major problem that is resistant to treatment in long COVID syndrome, compounded by fatigue and malaise.

References

1.   NHS England. Your COVID Recovery. After a stay on an intensive care unit. Available from: https://www.yourcovidrecovery.nhs.uk/what-is-covid-19/after-a-stay-on-icu/.

2.   Tansey CM, Louie M, Loeb M. One-year outcomes and health care utilization in survivors of severe acute respiratory syndrome. *Arch Intern Med* 2007; 167: 1312–20.

3.   Bienvenu OJ, Friedman LA, Colantuoni E, *et al.* Psychiatric symptoms after acute respiratory distress syndrome: a 5-year longitudinal study. *Intensive Care Med* 2018; 44: 38–47.

4.   Pandharipande PP, Girard TD, Jackson JC, *et al.* Long-term cognitive impairment after critical illness. *N Engl J Med* 2013; 369: 1306–16.

5.   Wilson JE, Mart MF, Cunningham C, *et al.* Delirium. *Nat Rev Dis Primers* 2020; 6: 90.

6.   Guillon A, Laurent E, Godillon L, *et al.* Long-term mortality of elderly patients after intensive care unit admission for COVID-19. *Intensive Care Med* 2021; 47: 710–2.

7.   McCue C, Cowan R, Quasim T, *et al.* Long term outcomes of critically ill COVID-19 pneumonia patients: early learning. *Intensive Care Med* 2021; 47: 240–1.

Chapter 7

Risk factors for developing long COVID syndrome

Introduction

Both COVID-19 and long COVID syndrome are still relatively new entities since COVID-19 first emerged, and their risk factors remain poorly defined. Our present knowledge is based primarily on patients' self-reported data and information on symptoms gathered via online apps. Further, the wide range of symptoms of long COVID syndrome makes statistical analyses even more complex.

Type and number of symptoms in early infection

Patients who experience more than five symptoms in the first week of COVID-19 illness have a threefold increased risk of developing long COVID syndrome (odds ratio 3.53), regardless of sex and age group. The commonest symptoms that contribute to a higher risk of long COVID syndrome include fatigue, headache, dyspnoea, voice hoarseness and myalgia.

Illness severity during acute infection

According to a very recent Swiss study, severe critical illness during acute infection was a risk factor for developing long COVID syndrome (odds ratio 4.0).

Age

The incidence of long COVID syndrome at 4 weeks post-infection was reported to be higher with increasing age (9.9% risk in those aged 18–49 years vs. 21.9% in those aged ≥70 years).

The prevalence of long COVID syndrome in children is still debatable. Although the incidence and severity have been found to be low in children, the prevalence of long COVID syndrome in those affected differed across studies. A Russian study reported that a quarter of children experienced persistent symptoms months after hospitalisation with COVID-19, with 1 in 10 having multisystem involvement. By contrast, a Swiss study, examining antibody levels in children, estimated a very low prevalence of long COVID syndrome in children and adolescents, with 9–10% and 2–4% having persistent symptoms for at least 4 weeks and more than 12 weeks, respectively.

Gender

Long COVID syndrome has been found to be commoner in women (14.5%) than in men (9.5%) at 4 weeks post-acute COVID illness (particularly in younger age groups). This correlates with the fact that women are 50% more likely to develop long COVID syndrome than men. By contrast, men are more likely to be hospitalised and have a higher risk of mortality in acute COVID than women. Similar results were found in a Swiss population-based cohort study (43% in women vs. 31.5% in men).

The same Swiss study (mentioned above) further showed that women with pre-existing mental illness and cardiovascular risk factors have a higher risk of developing long COVID syndrome.

Socioeconomic status

Studies have shown that all socioeconomic classes carry a similar risk of developing long COVID syndrome.

High body mass index

According to researchers in the UK, long COVID syndrome is commoner in patients with increasing body mass index. In addition, a Swiss cohort study showed that obesity is a risk factor for long COVID syndrome in men (odds ratio 1.44), but not in women.

Other systemic illnesses associated with long COVID syndrome

Pre-existing asthma was found to be associated with an increased risk of long COVID syndrome, with symptoms lasting for >4 weeks (odds ratio 2.14). Further, one study found that a history of allergic disease in children represented a strong risk factor for long COVID syndrome.

Prediction models of long COVID syndrome

Increasing age (29.2%) and the number of symptoms during the first week of acute infection (16.3%) have been found to be strong predictors of long COVID syndrome. Another app-based prediction model targeting age, sex, body mass index and number of symptoms in the first week of acute COVID-19 identified >69% of patients who developed long COVID syndrome (sensitivity), while being 73% effective at avoiding false alarms (specificity). These models hold promise for the future, with the aim of providing education and interventional methods to high-risk patient populations, and thus minimising the burden of long COVID syndrome to society and the health care system.

Long COVID syndrome and symptom relapse

Patients with long COVID syndrome were found to have a higher risk of experiencing symptoms post-recovery of acute COVID-19 illness (16%), compared to those who did not have long COVID syndrome (8.4%).

Better awareness of risk factors for long COVID syndrome will help towards assessing the true impact of long COVID syndrome on health care resources, thus, in turn, enabling proper planning of appropriate health care delivery. Long COVID syndrome will be a major problem in the long term once the pandemic is under control — which is why all health and social care sectors should work together in recognising and rehabilitating patients suffering from long COVID syndrome.

Key Points

- The presence of more than five symptoms during acute COVID infection carries a threefold increased risk of developing long COVID syndrome.
- Long COVID syndrome is more prevalent in older age groups and in women.
- Models to predict higher risk of long COVID syndrome will help in better management of resource utilisation and health care delivery.

References

1. Sudre CH, Murray B, Varsavsky T, et al. Attributes and predictors of long COVID. Nat Med 2021; 27: 626–31.
2. COVID Symptom Study (2021). One in 20 people likely to suffer from 'long COVID', but who are they? Available from: https://covid.joinzoe.com/us-post/long-covid.
3. Gebhard CE, Sutsch C, Bengs S, et al. Sex- and gender-specific risk factors of post-COVID-19 syndrome: a population-based cohort study in Switzerland. doi: https://doi.org/10.1101/2021.06.30.21259757. Pre-print research available from: https://www.medrxiv.org/content/10.1101/2021.06.30.21259757v1.
4. Osmanov IM, Spiridonova E, Bobkova P, et al. Risk factors for long COVID in previously hospitalised children using the ISARIC global follow-up protocol: a prospective cohort study. Eur Respir J 2021. Online ahead of print. Available from: https://doi.org/10.1183/13993003.01341-2021.
5. Radtke T, Ulyte A, Puhan MA, et al. Long-term symptoms after SARS-CoV-2 infection in school children: population-based cohort with 6-months follow-up. doi: 10.1101/2021.05.16.21257255. Available from: https://www.medrxiv.org/content/10.1101/2021.05.16.21257255v1.full-text.
6. Sudre CH, Murray B, Varsavsky T, et al. Attributes and predictors of long-COVID: analysis of COVID cases and their symptoms collected by the COVID Symptoms Study App. doi: 10.1101/2020.10.19.20214494. Available from: https://www.medrxiv.org/content/10.1101/2020.10.19.20214494v2.

Chapter 8

Effects of long COVID syndrome on economy and society

Introduction

History has taught us the long-term economic damage that pandemics can inflict, as was the case with the plague and Spanish flu pandemics. While it is clear that the ongoing COVID-19 pandemic is having a significant effect on our economy, employment and society as a whole, causing a severe recession, we are yet to see the long-term economic and societal effects of the pandemic, as well as the effects of long COVID syndrome.

The magnitude of the recession as a result of the acute pandemic has been unprecedented. In the UK alone, the gross domestic product (GDP) declined by 9.8% in 2020, the steepest decline since records began and in over 300 years, as per published estimates. In the United States, COVID-19 has been the biggest threat to prosperity and well-being, and estimated to have cost over $16 trillion (as of October 2020).

In the UK, the government offered financial support through the furlough scheme to those who were in employment but could not actively be in work due to the COVID-19 pandemic, at an estimated cost of approximately £15 billion per month, which was just below the NHS budget per month for the country. Financial experts have predicted that the prolonged period of depressed economy and secular stagnation due to COVID-19 alone could linger for two decades or more. As governments focus on short-term mitigation and containment strategies, as well as on their costs, this chapter will focus on the effect of long COVID syndrome and its disastrous consequences on society.

'Long economic COVID'

An article in the *Financial Times* proposed that long COVID syndrome should refer not only to its impact on health, but also to its consequences on the economy. It described the threat of 'long economic COVID' with years of debility, in addition to deep recession. For this reason, it is important for stakeholders and policymakers to understand the impact of long COVID syndrome in real terms.

In the context of long COVID syndrome, it is estimated that there are approximately seven times as many survivors of severe COVID-19 disease as there are COVID-related deaths. Based on these calculations, long-term impairment due to long COVID syndrome would affect more than twice as many people as the number of deaths due to acute COVID-19 illness. Significant long-term health-related complications, including respiratory, cardiac and mental health problems, would be costly to the economy and strain the health care system.

Costs due to mental health impairment

An American study estimated a prevalence of 40% of symptoms of depression and anxiety as a result of long COVID syndrome in 2020 (compared with 11% in 2019), with associated costs of $20,000 per person per year, resulting in an overall loss of $16 trillion.

Costs due to disruption of children's education

The Wellcome Trust charity predicts that almost half of the world's student population have been affected by school closures, even at 1 year since the pandemic began. It further predicts worryingly that millions of girls in poorer countries may never return to school.

Costs on vital social issues

COVID-19 has led to significant costs related to many societal issues. For example, the Wellcome Trust charity predicts that 135 million more people will be pushed into poverty by 2030, and there will be 30% less investment in clean energy transition. A total of 255 million full-time jobs were lost in 2020 in terms of working hours, and women have been harder hit economically. In summary, the impact of COVID-19 on many facets of our society is already being felt.

Costs due to job losses

Job losses not only impact directly on the economy, but also affect morbidity and mortality rates. A study of workers in Pennsylvania showed that mortality rates were 10–15% higher among those who suffered job losses, compared to other workers. Younger people are more likely to lose their jobs, particularly impacting those in minority communities and especially those with lower levels of education.

An international cohort study on more than 3700 patients who had COVID-19 showed that 45.2% required a reduced work schedule at 6 months post-COVID-19 illness, compared to before the illness, and 22.3% were not in active work due to health problems.

Burden of long COVID syndrome

Compared to other natural calamities, COVID-19 presents a peculiar problem of not knowing when the pandemic will 'really' end! The effects of long COVID syndrome on health care resource utilisation and the economy are very difficult to predict. Previous studies on severe acute respiratory distress syndrome in young people have shown limitations to exercise capacity even up to 5 years post-illness. It is difficult to estimate the effects of long COVID syndrome on exercise tolerance. Even when the pandemic is declared to be over, the lasting burden of mental health problems, chronic pain and societal problems will still take a big toll on the economy.

Many specialists have started using the term 'syndemic', rather than 'pandemic', for COVID-19. 'Syndemic' refers to a number of pre-existing conditions, with emphasis on non-communicable diseases, as well as to socioeconomic, political, climatological and environmental parameters.

Delayed care and associated costs

An American report has quoted $30–65 billion of annual increase in costs due to deferred care as a result of the pandemic. It states that 40% of patients have had their hospital appointments cancelled and an extra 12% reported not having received care. Deferred care costs can vary, depending on the disease. For example, in cancer treatment or in the management of chronic obstructive pulmonary disease, even small delays can highly impact patient outcome.

Impact of abnormal sense of smell in long COVID syndrome

Anosmia (absent sense of smell) and hyposmia (reduced sense of smell) have received much attention as secondary sequelae of long COVID syndrome. These are reported to have significant effects on daily living and well-being. Parosmia (distorted sense of smell) is seen in up to 43% of COVID-19 patients, of whom 1 in 5 show no improvement after 6 months. An impaired sense of smell affects sufferers' appetite and food intake, as well as their mental health, in turn indirectly affecting health care resource utilisation and the economy.

Costs due to COVID-induced disability

In the UK, it is estimated that 1 in 5 patients hospitalised due to COVID-19 illness would develop a new disability after their discharge from hospital. American studies have also found similar results in non-hospitalised people affected by COVID-19. It is estimated that 30% of the burden directly related to the COVID-19 pandemic could be due to long-term COVID-induced disability, rather than due to death in acute illness.

Challenges in estimating costs

It is very difficult to estimate costs due to long COVID syndrome, given that it is still unclear whether the strategy of full vaccination would reduce the incidence of COVID-19. A Member of Parliament chairing the All-Party Parliamentary Group on Coronavirus quoted in the news that long COVID syndrome could cost the UK alone £2.5 billion per year.

Long COVID syndrome leads to a range of indirect costs related to health care, mental well-being, societal problems and the economy. It is very difficult to perform accurate costing, due to hidden costs that can be easily missed in the calculation process.

Tackling long COVID syndrome in the UK's National Health Service

In December 2020, the NHS announced the opening of 69 specialist centres to treat long COVID syndrome patients, with the provision of £10 million. This was expanded to 83 clinics across England, with a cost of £24 million, by April 2021, and the need for such facilities is predicted to increase in the future. The UK government has provided £50 million for research on long COVID syndrome. In June 2021, the NHS announced specialist services for children and young people, as part of expansion plans for long COVID syndrome care costing £100 million. It was also announced that £30 million would be provided for enhanced services in primary care to improve identification, assessment and management of long COVID syndrome in patients presenting to their primary care physicians. It is understood that these budget needs will significantly increase in the near future.

Key Points

- 'Long economic COVID' refers to the impact of COVID-19 on the long-term economy and society.
- There are seven times more survivors of COVID-19 than those who died as a result of severe COVID-19; this puts high pressure on the resources and budgeting in terms of long-term health and social care management.
- The COVID 'syndemic' refers to the combination of pre-existing conditions, including non-communicable diseases, and socioeconomic, political, climatological and environmental parameters.
- One in five patients with COVID-19 develops a new disability after discharge from hospital; 30% of the economic burden of COVID-19 illness overall is due to COVID-induced disability.
- NHS costs due to long COVID syndrome are estimated to be around £2.5 billion per year.

References

1. Jorda O, Singh SR, Taylor AM. The long economic hangover of pandemics. *Finance & Development* 2020; 57: 12–5.

2. Cutler DM, Summers LH. The COVID-19 pandemic and the $16 trillion virus. *JAMA* 2020; 324: 1495–6.

3. Gathergood J. The economy after COVID-19. University of Nottingham. Available from: https://www.nottingham.ac.uk/vision/vision-economy-after-covid-19.

4. Harai D, Keep M, Brien P (2021). Coronavirus: economic impact. UK Parliament. House of Commons Library. Available from: https://commonslibrary.parliament.uk/research-briefings/cbp-8866/.

5. Coe EH, Enomoto K, Finn P, Stenson J, Weber K (2020). Understanding the hidden costs of COVID-19's potential impact on US healthcare. McKinsey & Company. Available from: https://www.mckinsey.com/industries/healthcare-systems-and-services/our-insights/understanding-the-hidden-costs-of-covid-19s-potential-impact-on-us-healthcare.

6. The British Academy (2021). The COVID decade: understanding the long-term societal impacts of COVID-19. The British Academy, London. doi: doi.org/10.5871/bac19stf/9780856726583.001. Available from: https://www.thebritishacademy.ac.uk/documents/3238/COVID-decade-understanding-long-term-societal-impacts-COVID-19.pdf.

7. Davis HE, Assaf GS, McCorkell L, *et al*. Characterizing long COVID in an international cohort: 7 months of symptoms and their impact. doi: https://doi.org/10.1101/2020.12.24.20248802. Available from: https://www.medrxiv.org/content/10.1101/2020.12.24.20248802v3.

8. Hopkins C, Watson DLB, Kelly C, *et al*. Managing long COVID: don't overlook olfactory dysfunction. *BMJ* 2020; 370: m3736.

9. Jones H (2021). Long COVID 'could cost UK around £2,500,000,000 a year'. Metro. Available from: https://metro.co.uk/2021/02/10/long-covid-could-cost-uk-around-2500000000-a-year-14050266/.

10. Briggs A, Vassall A. Count the cost of disability caused by COVID-19. *Nature* 2021; 593: 502–5.

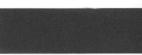

Section II

Symptoms and investigations

Chapter 9

Respiratory problems

Introduction

It is well known that SARS-CoV-2 affects the respiratory system to a significant extent, causing serious morbidities in the long term. Even studies that were reported early in the pandemic found that respiratory symptoms can last for many months after the initial illness.

Aetiopathogenesis of respiratory problems

SARS-CoV-2 targets alveolar epithelial cells. Based on what is already known in other respiratory illnesses, damage to these cells leads to pulmonary fibrosis, with ensuing chronic lung problems.

Cytokine storm can cause dysregulated repair, as well as fibrosis, after the initial inflammatory changes. In severe cases of COVID-19, lung scarring and resulting interstitial lung disease lead to breathlessness and malaise that can last long term.

Acute COVID-19 and lung damage

Many patients who have suffered from COVID-19 illness recover fully; however, a number of COVID-19 patients also have long-term lung damage. The latter group comprises patients with a 'stormy' course of acute illness requiring oxygen support, including also, in a few cases, mechanical ventilation, tracheostomy, high-flow oscillatory ventilation and extracorporeal membrane oxygenation. Compared to other causes of acute respiratory distress syndrome, COVID-19 presents unique challenges with multisystem involvement, severe cytokine storm/inflammatory responses and coagulation-related complications.

Post-mortem studies have shown characteristic features of the exudative and proliferative phases of diffuse alveolar damage in patients who had COVID-19 infection, including capillary congestion, necrotic lung cells, hyaline membranes, interstitial and intra-alveolar oedema, cellular changes and platelet-fibrin thrombi. Inflammatory infiltrates were shown to be composed of macrophages and lymphocytes. In acute stages, the viral particles were predominantly found in pneumocytes.

Studies using high-resolution computed tomography (CT) have described bilateral consolidation, subpleural line and ground-glass opacities in patients with COVID-19. Compared to other respiratory distress conditions, acute stages of COVID-19 illness have been found to be resistant to treatment due to problems with lung compliance and fibrosis. A greater degree of thrombogenic inflammation has also been noted in these patients.

Long COVID syndrome and the lungs

In an Italian study, the first on long COVID syndrome in patients who had COVID-19 and were followed up for months in the outpatient clinic, shortness of breath (dyspnoea) was noted in 43% of patients, and chest pain in 21.7%. In these patients, 53.1% also reported the symptom of fatigue. Both fatigue and shortness of breath were the commonest symptoms in this population.

In a 6-month follow-up study of COVID-19 patients discharged from Wuhan, China, pulmonary function tests and high-resolution chest CT were used to study the respiratory effects in greater detail. Results showed a significant risk of decreased lung diffusion capacity, which was worse in patients who required ventilatory support at the time of hospitalisation (56%). There was also a significantly higher incidence of lung changes found on CT in patients who required ventilation (41–45%). Ground-glass opacity was the commonest CT finding at follow-up.

A similar 3-month follow-up study from Belgium of COVID-19 patients reported that 25% had dyspnoea, 35% had fatigue and 45% had decreased lung diffusion capacity, while 17% had lung parenchymal changes and 21% had signs of fibrosis on high-resolution chest CT. The number of days in the intensive care unit correlated with persistent lesions on CT. Intubation also was found to be associated with fibrosis on CT. However, the severity of lung damage on CT imaging or pulmonary function tests was not predictive of dyspnoea or fatigue.

In another follow-up study of non-ventilated patients from Wuhan, dyspnoea scores and exercise capacity improved over time at 12 months after COVID-19 illness. However, a subgroup of patients had persistent physiological and radiological changes. Median lung diffusion capacity was 77% of predicted at 3 months after discharge from hospital and improved to 88% of predicted at 12 months after hospital discharge. Radiological changes persisted in 24% of patients at 12 months.

Even in dyspnoeic patients with long COVID syndrome who had normal or near-normal CT imaging, studies using hyperpolarised xenon (^{129}Xe) magnetic resonance imaging (MRI) showed limitation to alveolar-capillary diffusion at 3 months after COVID-19 illness.

Respiratory signs and symptoms in long COVID syndrome

The respiratory signs and symptoms in long COVID syndrome are outlined in ■ Table 9.1 overleaf.

Table 9.1. Respiratory signs and symptoms in long COVID syndrome.

- Shortness of breath
- Cough
- Chest tightness or pain
- Increased respiratory rate
- Shallow breathing
- Difficulty in breathing
- Decreased oxygen saturation on pulse oximetry
- Extreme tiredness due to breathlessness
- Inability to exercise or perform simple activities due to respiratory distress
- Sore throat

Presentation of multiple comorbidities

Shortness of breath can be due to coexisting cardiac and respiratory causes, leading to difficulty in diagnosing and treating sufferers of long COVID syndrome with dyspnoea. Early appropriate investigation can help in understanding the exact causes and targeting treatment appropriately.

Anxiety is common in long COVID syndrome and can be exacerbated by fatigue and sleep problems. Anxiety can present with dysfunctional breathing, palpitations and a vicious cycle of decreased activity and deconditioning of all muscles. In many patients, this can be superimposed by symptoms related to respiratory and cardiac comorbidities, making these individuals more prone to persistence of long COVID symptoms. A holistic approach based on a biopsychosocial model is important, while serious/sinister symptoms are appropriately investigated and explained to the patient.

Key Points

- COVID-19 affects the respiratory system to a significant extent and can persist for months post-illness.
- Shortness of breath, cough and chest tightness or chest pain are common persistent respiratory symptoms in long COVID syndrome.
- Lung compliance is reduced, with persistent fibrosis, in long COVID syndrome.
- Appropriate investigations are important to rule out serious treatable respiratory causes.

References

1. Fraser E. Long term respiratory complications of Covid-19. *BMJ* 2020; 370: m3001.

2. Carsana, Sonzogni A, Nasr A, *et al.* Pulmonary post-mortem findings in a series of northern Italy: a two centre descriptive study. *Lancet Infect Dis* 2020; 20: 1135–40.

3. Hayes JP. Considering the long-term respiratory effects of Covid-19. *Occup Med* (Lond) 2021; 71: 325–7.

4. Carfi A, Bernabei R, Landi F, *et al.* Persistent symptoms in patients after acute COVID-19. *JAMA* 2020; 324: 603–5.

5. Huang C, Huang L, Wang Y, *et al.* 6-month consequences of COVID-19 in patients discharged from hospital: a cohort study. *Lancet* 2021; 397: 220–32.

6. Froidure A, Mahsouli A, Liistro G, *et al.* Integrative respiratory follow-up of severe COVID-19 reveals common functional and lung imaging sequelae. *Respir Med* 2021; 181: 106383.

7. Wu X, Liu X, Zhou Y, *et al.* 3-month, 6-month, 9-month and 12-month respiratory outcomes in patients following COVID-19 related hospitalisation: a prospective study. *Lancet Respir Med* 2021; 9: 747–54.

8. Grist JT, Chen M, Collier GJ, *et al.* Hyperpolarised ^{129}Xe MRI abnormalities in dyspneic participants 3 months after COVID-19 pneunonia: preliminary results. *Radiology* 2021; 301: E353–60.

Chapter 10

Cardiovascular problems

Introduction

SARS-CoV-2 causes significant damage to the heart that can last beyond the recovery period and become persistent as part of long COVID syndrome. Heart failure and life-threatening arrhythmias are seen in COVID-19 illness. It is known that SARS-CoV-2 infection leads to vascular dysfunction, immunological and inflammatory responses, coagulation abnormalities and thrombosis. The resultant damage can even affect COVID-19 patients lifelong.

Aetiopathogenesis of cardiovascular problems

During acute infection, SARS-CoV-2 affects the heart by causing inflammatory damage. Elevated troponin levels and heart failure have been noted in critically ill patients. Proposed mechanisms of cardiac injury include inflammatory plaque rupture, thrombosis, cardiac stress, angiotensin-converting enzyme 2 (ACE2) receptor-mediated endotheliitis, interstitial mononuclear inflammation and myocarditis.

Further, increased right ventricular load due to pulmonary embolism or pneumonia leads to cardiac strain and injury. At a vascular level, fibrin thrombi are present in alveolar capillaries, with endothelial inflammation and thrombosis, leading to microvascular damage. Accelerated atherosclerosis and thromboembolic disease increase the afterload.

Microvascular injury leads to impaired myocardial flow reserve and causes cellular damage. COVID-19-related sepsis causes hypotension, hypoxia and shock, leading to myocardial injury.

SARS-CoV-2 infection induces increased expression of ACE2 on cardiomyocytes. It has been suggested that the virus exerts its cardiovascular effects through interaction between the viral spike (S) protein and ACE2, which triggers viral entry into host cells.

Acute COVID-19 and cardiac damage

A number of patients with COVID-19 who present with chest pain are diagnosed with acute coronary syndrome, as confirmed by raised troponin levels and ST segment elevation on the electrocardiogram (ECG). An early study from Germany in 2020 showed that 78% of COVID-19-infected patients had cardiac involvement, including 60% with myocardial inflammation, based on magnetic resonance imaging (MRI) of the heart. The authors found that these results were independent of pre-existing conditions, severity and overall course of the illness.

A study published in the *European Heart Journal* on 1216 COVID-19 patients from 69 countries found that over half of the patients (55%) had abnormalities on echocardiography following SARS-CoV-2 infection. In this study, 1 in 7 patients had severe problems affecting their survival and recovery.

An American study using transthoracic echocardiography in hospitalised patients with acute COVID-19 showed that nearly 35% had a left ventricular ejection fraction of <50%. These patients remained at high risk of myocardial injury, even after their discharge from hospital.

COVID-19 is associated with coagulation abnormalities leading to thromboembolic events, with elevated D-dimer levels. Hypercoagulable states lead to serious thrombotic events and stroke in susceptible patients.

Renal damage leading to cardiorenal syndrome also results in cardiac injury.

Long COVID syndrome and the heart

It has been found that about 80% of patients with severe COVID-19 illness have cardiac involvement, with nearly 25% having myocardial inflammation at 3 months after diagnosis.

Viral myocarditis leads to heart failure, atrial and ventricular arrhythmias, impaired exercise tolerance and even sudden cardiac death.

A Spanish study on patients who had confirmed SARS-CoV-2 infection found that, at 10 weeks post-illness, 42% had chest pain, dyspnoea or palpitations, 50% had ECG abnormalities, 75% had cardiac MRI abnormalities, 3% had pericarditis, 26% had myocarditis and 11% had both pericarditis and myocarditis.

Long COVID syndrome and the vascular system

Endothelial cells are a direct target of SARS-CoV-2, as demonstrated by endothelial inflammation in histological studies.

Cardiovascular signs and symptoms in long COVID syndrome

Cardiovascular signs and symptoms in long COVID syndrome are outlined in ■ Table 10.1 overleaf.

Table 10.1. Cardiovascular signs and symptoms in long COVID syndrome.

- Chest tightness or pain
- Dyspnoea or shortness of breath (worse on lying down or on exertion)
- Palpitations
- Cough
- Dizziness
- Pedal oedema
- Postural hypotension and tachycardia
- Fatigue
- Nausea
- Sweating
- Arrhythmias on ECG

Postural hypotension

Postural orthostatic tachycardia syndrome (POTS) has been reported as part of long COVID syndrome. Autonomic nervous system imbalance causes dysregulation of heart rate and blood flow. Affected patients experience a fast heart rate, palpitations and light-headedness, and if persistent, fatigue and brain fog.

Cardiovascular effects of antiviral medications

A number of antiviral medications have been found to have cardiac effects. Hydroxychloroquine (blocks viral entry) and azithromycin (macrolide antibiotic) can induce prolonged QT interval. Antiviral drug combinations such as lopinavir-ritonavir cause atrioventricular block. Tocilizumab, an interleukin 6 (IL-6) inhibitor, causes high blood pressure.

Key Points

- Severe COVID-19 causes cardiac damage (80%) that can persist for many months or longer; about 25% of patients remain symptomatic after 3 months.
- One in seven COVID-19 patients have long-term cardiac problems affecting their survival and recovery.
- Vascular dysfunction, inflammatory damage and thrombotic changes have been proposed as underlying mechanisms leading to cardiac sequelae.
- Postural hypotension causes symptoms in long COVID syndrome.

References

1. Puntmann VO, Carerj ML, Wieters I. Outcomes of cardiovascular magnetic resonance imaging in patients recently recovered from coronavirus disease 2019 (COVID-19). *JAMA Cardiol* 2020; 5: 1265–73.
2. Dweck MR, Bularga A, Hahn RT, *et al*. Global evaluation of echocardiography in patients with COVID-19. *Eur Heart J Cardiovasc Imaging* 2020; 21: 949–58.
3. Nishiga M, Wang DW, Han Y, *et al*. COVID-19 and cardiovascular disease: from basic mechanisms to clinical perspectives. *Nat Rev Cardiol* 2020; 17: 543–58.
4. Becker RC. Anticipating the long-term cardiovascular effects of COVID-19. *J Thromb Thrombolysis* 2020; 50: 512–24.
5. Jain SS, Liu Q, Raikhelkar J, *et al*. Indications for and findings on transthoracic echocardiography in COVID-19. *J Am Soc Echocardiogr* 2020; 33: 1278–84.
6. Eiros R, Barreiro-Perez M, Martin-Garcia, et al. Pericarditis and myocarditis long after SARS-CoV-2 infection: a cross-sectional descriptive study in health-care workers. 2020 July. Available from: https://www.medrxiv.org/content/10.1101/2020.07.12.20151316v1.

Chapter 11

Neurological problems

Introduction

It is now well established that COVID-19 illness affects the brain and neurological system significantly. Even early in the pandemic, the effects of the illness on the neurological system were obvious, with patients presenting with symptoms of anosmia (loss of smell sensation), stroke and cognitive and psychological impairment. Many intensive care patients with COVID-19 suffered from significant delirium, one of the risk factors for developing long COVID syndrome.

Incidence of neurological problems in long COVID syndrome

It is estimated overall that 30–50% of patients hospitalised with COVID-19 have illness-related neurological issues. In addition, there is a reported incidence of dizziness and headache of 17% and 13%, respectively.

In a retrospective study using data on more than 230,000 COVID-19 patients from the United States, the incidence of a neurological or psychiatric diagnosis in the 6 months following COVID-19 diagnosis was 33.62%. This incidence was increased (46.42%) for patients who had been admitted to the intensive care unit. Further data showed the incidence of ischaemic stroke, dementia and anxiety disorder was 2.10%, 0.67% and 17.39%, respectively, in the entire cohort of patients in the 6 months from their COVID-19 diagnosis. An Italian study also reported similar findings of neurological abnormalities at 6 months, with an incidence of 37.4%.

Neurological problems, including stroke and brain damage, lead to long-term problems, thus contributing to the persistence of long COVID syndrome.

Aetiopathogenesis of nervous system involvement

SARS-CoV-2 is a neurotropic virus. The olfactory bulb has been proposed as its route of entry into the brain, which could explain the occurrence of anosmia. Other suggested routes into the brain include viraemia and via infected white blood cells. SARS-CoV-2 has been shown to replicate in nerve cells. The angiotensin-converting enzyme 2 (ACE2) receptor, to which the virus binds, has been found in the brain vascular endothelium and smooth muscle. Elevated cytokine expression and macrophage infiltration are also found in affected tissues.

Coagulopathy secondary to the cytokine storm and inflammatory reactions could explain the occurrence of cerebrovascular disease in COVID-19 illness. Stroke due to COVID-19 is accompanied by low platelet counts and raised D-dimer and C-reactive protein (CRP) levels.

Neurological signs and symptoms in long COVID syndrome

Neurological symptoms include weakness, fatigue, muscle aches and pain, headache, dizziness, confusion, memory problems, seizures, delirium and stroke. Altered smell and taste sensations can persist in long COVID syndrome. The commonest symptoms reported are fatigue (77%), post-exertional malaise (72%) and cognitive dysfunction (55%).

Neurological signs and symptoms in long COVID syndrome are outlined in ■ Table 11.1 overleaf.

Table 11.1. Neurological signs and symptoms in long COVID syndrome.

- Brain fog
- Difficulty to concentrate
- Memory problems
- Cognitive impairment
- Fatigue
- Post-exertional malaise
- Chronic pain
- Generalised weakness
- Headache
- Loss of smell and/or taste
- Delirium

Classification of neurological involvement

Neurological involvement has been categorised as follows:

- Damage limited to epithelial cells of the nose/mouth.
- Inflammatory response and blood clots leading to stroke.
- Explosive cytokine storm damaging the blood-brain barrier.

Brain fog

'Brain fog' is a term used to describe memory and concentration problems that are seen in many functional pain syndromes such as fibromyalgia. Unfortunately, brain fog is commonly experienced by patients with persistent long COVID syndrome, including those who were previously physically active before COVID-19 illness. Brain fog leads to loss of the affected individual's identity within their family, as well as their role in society, and negatively impacts their job performance. Poor awareness of these symptoms among health care professionals and families, as well as their work colleagues, can lead to increased distress and frustration.

Studies have shown that 85% of patients with long COVID syndrome reported suffering from brain fog or cognitive dysfunction. The commonest symptoms of brain fog include poor concentration (75%) and difficulty in thinking (65%). A survey conducted by the Royal College of General Practitioners presented to the UK Parliament reported an incidence of headache, brain fog and dizziness of 55%, 46% and 92%, respectively.

Stroke in COVID-19 illness

Stroke has been reported in patients with COVID-19, including those who had mild respiratory involvement. The incidence of stroke in acute illness is reported to be 2–6% among hospitalised patients.

Encephalitis

The presence of SARS-CoV-2 in the cerebrospinal fluid suggests that it could directly infect the brain. Further, immune-mediated encephalitis is also common.

Early studies reported variable incidences of encephalopathy, ranging from 7% in a study from Wuhan, China, to 69% in a French study.

Acute disseminated encephalomyelitis has been described in COVID-19 illness, with multifocal demyelination presenting with focal neurological symptoms.

Complications from intensive care stay

It is well known that 20–40% of intensive care patients experience delirium — a large proportion of whom are those requiring ventilation support — and this was the same even before the COVID-19 pandemic. COVID-19 can significantly worsen neurological symptoms and outcomes. Non-specific neurological symptoms are also present in COVID-19 illness due to critical care neuropathy and hypoxic brain damage. Drug side effects, positional neuropathies, hypercoagulable states and acute neuropathies can occur in these patients, further exacerbating persistent neurological presentations.

Mental health problems

It has been reported that 31% of patients with acute COVID-19 illness have altered mental status and 8% have psychosis. Cognitive impairment is seen in patients with acute COVID-19 illness, as well as in those with long COVID syndrome.

Changes in personality, behaviour, cognition and level of consciousness have also been reported in patients with long COVID syndrome. For more details on mental health problems, see Chapter 13.

Sleep problems

Changes in sleep pattern and difficulty sleeping are associated with long COVID syndrome, even months following acute infection. In a UK survey of COVID-19 patients carried out by the Royal College of General Practitioners, it was found that 76% of patients had sleep disorders or mood problems.

Peripheral nerve and muscle problems

Guillain-Barré syndrome has been reported in COVID-19 illness. Myopathy and neuropathy have been found to occur in long COVID syndrome, especially in patients who had prolonged intensive care stay. Chronic pain is a known problem in long COVID syndrome. For more details on pain in long COVID syndrome, see Chapter 12.

Key Points

- **More than 30% of patients with COVID-19 develop neurological problems; this is significantly worse in hospitalised patients.**
- **Fatigue (77%), post-exertional malaise (72%) and cognitive impairment (55%) are commonly reported symptoms in long COVID syndrome.**
- **Patients with long COVID syndrome experience brain fog, cognitive dysfunction and poor concentration.**
- **Sleep is affected in over 75% of patients with COVID-19 illness.**

References

1. Weir K. How COVID-19 attacks the brain. *Monitor on Psychology* 2020; 51: 20.

2. Ellul MA, Benjamin L, Singh B, *et al.* Neurological associations of COVID-19. *Lancet* 2020; 19: 767–83.

3. Davis HE, Assaf GS, McCorkell L, *et al.* Characterizing long COVID in an international cohort: 7 months of symptoms and their impact. Available from: https://www.medrxiv.org/content/10.1101/2020.12.24.20248802v3.

4. Pilotto A, Cristillo V, Piccinelli SC, *et al.* COVID-19 severity impacts on long-term neurological manifestation after hospitalisation. Available from: https://www.medrxiv.org/content/10.1101/2020.12.27.20248903v1.full-text.

5. Royal College of General Practitioners — Written evidence (COV0051). Ongoing or persistent symptoms of Covid-19 (long COVID). Available from: https://committees.parliament.uk/writtenevidence/12976/pdf/.

6. Taquet M, Geddes JR, Husain M, *et al.* 6-month neurological and psychiatric outcomes in 236379 survivors of COVID-19: a retrospective cohort study using electronic health records. *Lancet* 2021; 8: 416–27.

Chapter 12

Pain problems

Introduction

Chronic persistent pain and fatigue are two important problems that can persist for many months post-COVID-19 illness, hindering patient recovery. Chronic pain can be nociplastic in nature (i.e. characterised by abnormal perception of pain signals) and can cause psychological distress and social/occupational problems.

Chronic pain in long COVID syndrome

The REACT-2 (REal-time Assessment of Community Transmission-2) study from Imperial College London, assessed more than half a million patients affected by COVID-19 in the long term. At 12 weeks post-acute illness, more than one in three patients reported at least one symptom of long COVID syndrome. The authors categorised the symptoms into two groups:

- Group 1: tiredness as the predominating symptom — muscle aches and sleep problems.
- Group 2: respiratory and related symptoms — shortness of breath and chest pain.

Tiredness and pain are the two more commonly reported symptoms by patients with long COVID syndrome.

Clauw *et al* have proposed three categories of causative factors for chronic pain problems:

- Post-viral syndrome or virus-associated organ damage.
- Exacerbation of pre-existing pain due to physical or mental health problems.
- New chronic pain in those NOT affected by COVID-19, but due to the presence of risk factors (poor sleep, inactivity, fear, anxiety and depression).

For the purpose of this chapter, only the first category will be considered where chronic pain is directly associated with long COVID syndrome; an overlap with other conditions is undoubtedly inevitable.

Aetiopathogenesis of pain problems in long COVID syndrome

Various theories have been proposed, including:

- SARS-CoV-2 directly affecting neurons, thus causing pain (axonal polyneuropathy).
- Cytokine storm and immune dysregulation, causing neuronal-mediated changes.
- Thrombotic coagulation problems in the microvasculature.
- Stroke, seizures and encephalitis, causing long-term pain problems.
- Cranial neuropathies.
- Hospital and intensive care admission causing long-term pain problems.
- Multiple medications and their long-term side effects.
- Long COVID syndrome-related comorbidities causing pain syndrome.
- Psychological and sleep problems worsening pain presentation.
- Muscle deconditioning-related pain problems.

An early study from Wuhan, China, showed that COVID-19 patients with skeletal muscle injury had higher levels of creatine kinase, as well as higher neutrophil counts, lower lymphocyte counts and higher C-reactive protein and D-dimer levels. According to this study, 36.4% of patients had neurological involvement.

SARS-CoV-2 infection, through binding to the angiotensin-converting enzyme 2 (ACE2) receptor, identified as the functional receptor for the coronavirus, has been shown to affect the nervous system and skeletal muscles. Therefore, this could explain the neurological manifestations and pain problems seen in patients with long COVID syndrome.

Risk factors for chronic pain in COVID-19 illness

Kemp *et al* have proposed that those who survive critical illness with COVID-19 are at high risk of developing chronic pain in the presence of the following risk factors:

- Rehabilitation challenges (diverted resources, fatigue).
- Mental health burden (post-traumatic stress disorder, psychological issues).
- Neurological insult (neurotropism, immune response).
- Intensive care-specific factors (ventilation, immobility, medications, proning).
- At-risk population groups (elderly, individuals with comorbidities).
- High risk of acute pain (painful symptoms, procedural pain).

Pain presentations and sequelae in long COVID syndrome

Pain presentations and sequelae in long COVID syndrome are outlined in ■ Table 12.1 overleaf.

Table 12.1. Pain in long COVID syndrome.
■ Widespread pain
■ Dysaesthesia, allodynia, hyperalgesia
■ Neuropathic pain sensations, pins and needles, numbness
■ Joint pain
■ Chest pain
■ Myalgia, weakness, stiffness
■ Abdominal pain
■ Sore throat
■ Headache, earache, tinnitus
■ Fatigue, tiredness
■ Sleep problems
■ Lack of energy
■ Nausea and vomiting, loss of appetite
■ Inability to perform simple activities
■ Inability to concentrate, brain fog, memory problems
■ Medication-related side effects

Neurological conditions causing persistent pain in long COVID syndrome

Lengthy stays in intensive care can lead to critical illness myopathy and neuropathy, which, in turn, can cause persistent pain in COVID-19 patients. Further, COVID-19 can cause strokes, seizures, hypoxic sequelae, multiorgan failure-related neuropathy and Guillain-Barré syndrome — all of which can complicate the presentation of patients with long COVID syndrome by causing long-term pain.

Neuropathic pain in long COVID syndrome

Neuropathic pain, characterised by allodynia, dysaesthesia and a pins and needles sensation, is a common presentation in patients with long COVID syndrome. There is evidence of COVID-related nerve damage leading to pain in long COVID syndrome. A corneal confocal microscopy study has shown small nerve fibre loss and increased dendritic cell density, suggesting neurological insult and damage, in patients with long COVID syndrome. The authors used the pain scoring systems, Douleur Neuropathique 4 (DN4) and Fibromyalgia Questionnaire, to identify and determine the severity of nerve injury, and thus neuropathic pain.

A review article on the role of imaging in peripheral nerve injury has demonstrated its benefit in post-COVID-19 illness. Imaging can help characterise nerve abnormalities, identify the site and severity of nerve damage and elucidate the mechanisms of injury. The differential diagnosis of peripheral nerve injury in this situation includes post-infectious inflammatory neuropathy, prone position-related injury, compression injury, systemic neuropathy and nerve entrapment secondary to haematoma.

Mood, fatigue and pain

Chronic pain is the result of a vicious pain cycle — pain causes stiffness, which itself causes behavioural and emotional problems, in turn, leading to persistence of pain. Unless the vicious cycle is broken through health education and appropriate interventions, it can lead to a downhill spiral of worsening health, significantly impairing quality of life.

Exacerbation of chronic pain due to disruption of services

The provision of regular medical care has been significantly compromised during lockdown due to the COVID-19 pandemic. Many pain clinics in the UK were closed and health care staff resources were diverted to care provision for sick COVID-19 patients on wards and in emergency areas, as well as in intensive care units. As a result, patient access to chronic pain clinics and interventions was disrupted. Delayed access to basic pain management can lead to the persistence of chronic pain, even in individuals who have not had COVID-19. Poor psychological and mental well-being due to restrictions imposed by lockdown and an inability to access physical and social activities can also be contributing factors to the development of chronic pain.

Key Points

- Chronic pain is a distressing component of long COVID syndrome.
- Altered perception in pain signals and nerve damage occur due to a variety of reasons in COVID illness.
- Widespread pain and tiredness are common presentations in patients with long COVID syndrome.

References

1. Clauw DJ, Winfried H, Cohen SP, *et al*. Considering the potential for an increase in chronic pain after the COVID-19 pandemic. *Pain* 2020; 161: 1694–7.

2. Whitaker M, Elliott J, Chadeau-Hyam M, *et al*. Persistent symptoms following SARS-CoV-2 infection in a random community sample of 508,707 people. Available from: https://www.medrxiv.org/content/10.1101/2021.06.28.21259452v1.

3. Kemp HI, Corner E, Colvin LA. Chronic pain after COVID-19: implications for rehabilitation. *Br J Anaesth* 2020; 124: 436–40.

4. Mao L, Jin H, Wang M, *et al*. Neurologic manifestations of hospitalized patients with coronavirus disease 2019 in Wuhan, China. *JAMA Neurol* 2020; 77: 1–9.

5. Zhao Y, Zhao Z, Wang Y, *et al*. Single-cell RNA expression profiling of ACE2, the putative receptor for Wuhan 2019-nCov. *Am J Respir Crit Care Med* 2020; 202: 756–9.

6. Bitirgen G, Korkmaz C, Zamani A, *et al*. Corneal confocal microscopy identifies corneal nerve fibre loss and increased dendritic cells in patients with long COVID. *Br J Ophthalmol* 2021; 0: 1–7.

7. Fernandes CE, Franz CK, Ko JH, *et al*. Imaging review of peripheral nerve injuries in patients with COVID-19. *Radiology* 2021; 298: E117–30.

Chapter 13

Mental health problems

Introduction

The COVID-19 pandemic has caused a significant increase in psychological stress across populations worldwide. In the UK, the incidence of self-reported symptoms of depression in adults was 19% in June 2020, i.e. in the midst of the pandemic, compared to 10% before the pandemic. In the United States, the incidence of anxiety and depression increased from 11% before the pandemic to 42% in December 2020. The high mortality and morbidity rates due to COVID-19 illness, the economic problems that ensued and the complex rules of lockdown/social isolation have contributed to mental health exacerbation.

In addition to the acute illness itself and its sequelae, the continuing effects of long COVID syndrome have also significantly affected mental well-being. Fear and low mood can be exacerbated by the physical symptoms associated with long COVID syndrome. Restriction of activities and an inability to socialise are also barriers slowing patients' recovery from long COVID syndrome. Anxiety, depression and post-traumatic stress disorder (PTSD) have been reported in patients with long COVID syndrome, even many months after acute COVID-19 illness.

Aetiopathogenesis of mental health problems in long COVID syndrome

SARS-CoV-2 infection affects the brain directly, leading to psychiatric symptoms. Immunological/inflammatory dysregulation and cytokine storm also lead to mental health problems. It has been suggested that demyelination-type nerve damage can cause cognitive problems and psychosis. Psychological trauma due to stress and fear of illness can lead to the persistence of mental health problems in long COVID syndrome sufferers. Restricted mobility and comorbid conditions, as well as traumatic memories of acute illness and associated isolation, can all affect patients' mental well-being.

Epidemiology of mental health problems due to long COVID syndrome

A 6-month follow-up study of more than 2000 hospitalised patients diagnosed with COVID-19 in Wuhan, China, showed that 23% of patients had anxiety or depression, with 26% reporting sleep difficulties and 63% fatigue or muscle weakness.

In a recent 6-month follow-up study of nearly a quarter million people with COVID-19, the incidence of a neurological or psychiatric diagnosis after 6 months was 33.62%, of whom 12.84% had received their first such diagnosis. In patients treated in intensive care, the incidence of a diagnosis was 46.42%, of which the incidence of a first psychiatric diagnosis was 25.79%. The risks were higher in patients who had severe COVID-19 illness. In the same study, 23.98% of patients had mood or anxiety problems, 17.39% anxiety disorders and 5.42% insomnia problems.

Another study involving more than 1000 patients with COVID-19 discharged from hospital showed that 13.8% of patients screened positive for depression, and 10.5% for PTSD (at a median duration of 9 weeks after discharge).

A systematic review and meta-analysis of 50 studies comparing the prevalence of psychological burden in COVID-19 patients vs. the general population showed that the former group had a higher prevalence of psychological morbidities of 44%. In COVID-19 patients, the pooled prevalence of depression was 42% (compared to 24% in the general population) and of anxiety 37% (compared to 26% in the general population). The overall burden of post-traumatic stress syndrome was 96% (compared to 15% in the general population) and of poor sleep quality 82% (compared to 34% in the general population).

A study from the United States examined data of 62,354 patients diagnosed with COVID-19 across 54 health care organisations. The authors concluded that in patients with no previous psychiatric history, COVID-19 was associated with an increased incidence of psychiatric problems at 14–90 days post-diagnosis of COVID-19 (hazard ratio 2.1), with an increased risk of anxiety disorders, insomnia and dementia. The incidence of a first psychiatric diagnosis at 14–90 days post-COVID-19 diagnosis was 5.8% (compared to 2.5–3.4% in comparison cohorts). The incidence of a first diagnosis of dementia was 1.6% in people older than 65 years.

Signs and symptoms of mental health problems in long COVID syndrome

Signs and symptoms of mental health problems in long COVID syndrome are outlined in ■ Table 13.1 overleaf.

Table 13.1. Signs and symptoms of mental health problems in long COVID syndrome.

- Feeling anxious
- Low mood, depression
- Feeling upset, tearful
- Worries of future, job, family and finances
- Feeling hopeless
- Panic attacks
- Self-harm, suicidal feelings
- Post-traumatic stress disorder
- Persistent fear, flashbacks of hospital experiences
- Negative self-perception
- Feeling restless, change of routine
- Sleeplessness, poor-quality sleep
- Difficulty with finding pleasure in life
- Depersonalisation (feeling disconnected from mind or body)
- Feeling that life has changed significantly
- Psychotic feelings
- Delusion, hallucinations, speech problems
- Obsession about cleanliness
- Compulsion on accessing COVID-related news
- Paranoid feeling of leaving home due to fear

Mental health of families and carers

To have a family member suffering from long COVID syndrome is exhausting and frustrating for the patient's relatives and carers. Feeling helpless, not having a treatable diagnosis, fear of the future and loss of social status, including job loss, can lead to family distress, as well as strained family relations. Patients themselves with long COVID syndrome can lose their identity with respect to their social status, leading to frustration.

Key Points

- The incidence of anxiety and depression has increased significantly as a result of the COVID-19 pandemic.
- Sleep difficulties are a major problem among long COVID syndrome sufferers.
- PTSD has been reported in many patients suffering from long COVID syndrome.

References

1. Abbott A. COVID's mental-health toll: scientists track surge in depression. *Nature* 2021; 590: 194–5.
2. Taquet M, Geddes JR, Husain M, *et al.* 6-month neurological and psychiatric outcomes in 236,379 survivors of COVID-19: a retrospective cohort study using electronic health records. *Lancet Psychiatry* 2021; 8: 416–27.
3. Huang C, Huang L, Wang Y, *et al.* 6-month consequences of COVID-19 in patients discharged from hospital: a cohort study. *Lancet* 2021; 397: 220–32.
4. Naidu SB, Shah AJ, Saigal A, *et al.* The high mental health burden of 'long COVID' and its association with on-going physical and respiratory symptoms in all adults discharged from hospital. *Eur Respir J* 2021; 57: 2004364.
5. Krishnamoorthy Y, Nagarajan R, Saya GK, *et al.* Prevalence of psychological morbidities among general population, healthcare workers and COVID-19 patients amidst the COVID-19 pandemic: a systematic review and meta-analysis. *Psychiatry Res* 2020; 293: 113382.
6. Taquet M, Luciano S, Geddes JR, *et al.* Bidirectional associations between COVID-19 and psychiatric disorder: retrospective cohort studies of 62,354 COVID-19 cases in the USA. *Lancet Psychiatry* 2021; 8: 130–40.

Chapter 14

Taste and smell problems

Introduction

Loss of taste and smell sensations has been noted in acute COVID-19, presenting in the very early stages of illness, even before the onset of, or in the absence of, other symptoms of COVID-19. In a few patients, symptoms can persist, taking many months to recover. There are currently no prognostic data on long-term recovery from COVID-19. However, similar problems in other viral illnesses are known to persist even at 3 years post-acute illness.

Incidence of taste and smell problems

It has been estimated that about 1 in 10 patients with COVID-19 suffer from persistent taste and smell problems after their acute illness. Some studies have reported that in 1 in 20 patients with COVID-19, these problems can last up to 10 months post acute illness.

Using epidemiological and clinical data from 18 European hospitals, a multicentre study showed that the prevalence of olfactory dysfunction post-COVID-19 illness in the long term was 74.2% (85.9% mild, 6.9% moderate and 4.5% severe) and the prevalence of taste impairment was 45.8%.

Aetiopathology of taste and smell problems in long COVID syndrome

SARS-CoV-2 is a neurotropic virus with possible entry into the brain via the olfactory bulb, as proposed by some researchers, which would explain the occurrence of anosmia. However, other scientists have disagreed with this theory, suggesting that anosmia is the result of changes in olfactory physiology due to the involvement of the nasal epithelial cell lining near the olfactory bulb, rather than involving neural cells.

Bulk sequencing techniques have indicated other possible theories. Rather than neural cell involvement, it is possible that expression of angiotensin-converting enzyme 2 (ACE2) in sustentacular cells and olfactory bulb pericytes could result in anosmia. Animal studies have shown that non-neuronal cell types are affected in COVID-19, leading to the occurrence of anosmia.

Scientists from Italy have proposed yet another theory. They found that the loss of taste and smell is associated with increased levels of interleukin-6, which is an inflammatory cytokine. Another study, using post-mortem high-resolution magnetic resonance microscopy, showed leaky blood vessels around the olfactory bulbs.

Symptoms of smell and taste dysfunction

Patients with long COVID syndrome experience altered taste and smell of food; food can taste bland, salty or metallic. Taste and smell problems also affect appetite.

Parosmia (altered or distorted sense of taste and smell) can render a pleasant smell disgusting. Chemesthesis is a term used to describe the loss of taste sensation and the inability to detect chemically triggered sensations such as spiciness. Cacosmia is a type of parosmia where there is an unpleasant smell sensation. Phantosmia is when a patient smells odours that are not present (olfactory hallucinations).

All these conditions of altered sense of taste and smell have been reported in patients suffering from long COVID syndrome.

Objective measurements vs. self-reporting of symptoms of smell dysfunction

A meta-analysis of 24 studies involving >8000 patients found that 38.2% and 41% had taste and smell dysfunction, respectively. A higher prevalence of smell dysfunction was obtained through objective measurements than from self-reports, which suggests that many more patients could have had their diagnosis of COVID-19 missed through relying on self-reporting of symptoms.

Using the University of Pennsylvania Smell Identification Test (UPSIT), a specific 40-item psychophysical scoring system for smell dysfunction, researchers found that measurable smell dysfunction was extremely common (96%) in the acute phase of COVID-19 illness. About one-third of these patients continued to exhibit smell dysfunction even after 6–8 weeks of acute COVID-19 illness.

How long do symptoms of abnormal smell and taste sensations last?

In many patients affected by COVID-19 illness, taste and smell sensations recover within weeks. A 1-month follow-up study showed that 15.8% and 28.2% of patients with COVID-19 still had not recovered taste and smell sensations, respectively. However, some patients with long COVID syndrome have reported a very slow recovery, with some experiencing parosmia (unpleasant smell) and others anosmia that lasted for months.

A multicentre European study showed that 24.5% of patients did not recover olfaction 60 days after smell dysfunction onset. The mean duration of dysfunction was 21.6 (± 17.9) days, and 4.7% of anosmic/hyposmic patients did not recover olfaction at 6 months.

Consequences of taste and smell problems

An abnormal or absent sense of taste and smell is unpleasant and can lead to appetite loss. Absent taste and smell sensations can cause a sense of physical and social vulnerability, and consequently fear, thus impacting affected individuals both physically and psychosocially.

Key Points

- The prevalence of smell and taste dysfunction in COVID-19 illness is approximately 74% and 46%, respectively.
- One in 20 patients with smell and taste dysfunction might not recover even after 10 months post-acute COVID-19 illness.
- Sustentacular cells in the olfactory area have been suggested as possible targets of SARS-CoV-2; smell and taste dysfunction in long COVID syndrome could also be related to deranged interleukin-6 levels causing increased inflammation.
- The mean duration of olfactory dysfunction is 21.6 days, with the majority of affected patients recovering post-acute illness.

References

1. Your COVID recovery. Taste and smell. Available from: https://www.yourcovidrecovery.nhs.uk/managing-the-effects/effects-on-your-body/taste-and-smell/.
2. Lechien JR, Chiesa-Estomba CM, Beckers E, et al. Prevalence and 6-month recovery of olfactory dysfunction: a multicentre study of 1363 COVID-19 patients. J Intern Med 2021; 290: 451–61.
3. BBC News. Parosmia: The smells and tastes we still miss, long after Covid. Available from: https://www.bbc.co.uk/news/stories-55936729.

4.   Brann DH, Tsukahara T, Weinreb C, *et al.* Non-neuronal expression of SARS-CoV-2 entry genes in the olfactory system suggests mechanism underlying COVID-19-associated anosmia. *Sci Adv* 2020; 6: eabc5801.

5.   Cazzolla AP, Lovero R, Muzio LL, *et al.* Taste and smell disorders in COVID-19 patients: role of interleukin-6. *ACS Chem Neurosci* 2020; 11: 2774–81.

6.   Lee M, Perl DP, Nair G, *et al.* Microvascular injury in the brains of patients with Covid-19. *N Engl J Med* 2021; 384: 481–3.

7.   Marshall M. COVID's toll on smell and taste: what scientists know. *Nature* 2021; 589: 342–43.

8.   Agyeman AA, Chin KL, Landersdorfer CB, *et al.* Smell and taste dysfunction in patients with COVID-19: a systematic review and meta-analysis. *Mayo Clin Proc* 2020; 95: 1621–31.

9.   Moein ST, Hashemian SM, Tabarsi P, *et al.* Prevalence and reversibility of smell dysfunction measured psychophysically in a cohort of COVID-19 patients. *Int Forum Allergy Rhinol* 2020; 10: 1127–35.

10. Reiter ER, Coelho DH, Kons ZA, *et al.* Subjective smell and taste changes during the pandemic: short term recovery. *Am J Otolaryngol* 2020; 41: 102639.

Chapter 15

Other problems found in long COVID syndrome

Introduction

This chapter describes other symptoms with which patients affected by long COVID syndrome can present.

Prevalence

An online survey on long COVID syndrome involving 3762 patients with COVID-19 estimated the prevalence of 203 symptoms in ten organ systems and traced 66 symptoms for over 7 months. The authors found that these symptoms impacted the sufferers' life, work ability and performance and return to baseline health. During acute illness, the patients reported an average of 55.9 symptoms across an average of 9.1 organ systems. After 6 months, the commonest symptoms were fatigue, post-exertional malaise and cognitive dysfunction.

Other signs and symptoms in long COVID syndrome

Other signs and symptoms in long COVID syndrome are outlined in ■ Table 15.1 overleaf.

Table 15.1. Other signs and symptoms in long COVID syndrome.

- Extreme tiredness and fatigue
- Lack of energy
- Difficulty in performing simple tasks
- Brain fog
- Difficulty with concentration
- Memory problems
- Tinnitus
- Earache
- Feeling sick
- Diarrhoea, constipation, reflux
- Loss of appetite
- Fever
- Cough
- Sneezing, runny nose
- Sore throat
- Headaches
- Skin rashes
- Changes in menstrual cycles
- Chills, flushing, sweating
- Itching
- Dermatographia (light scratching causing raised red lines)
- COVID toe (swelling, colour change)
- Speech problems, slurring
- Hearing problems
- Visual symptoms, blurred vision
- Sexual dysfunction
- Bladder control problems

Fatigue and extreme tiredness in long COVID syndrome

A Canadian online survey found that 71.4% of patients with long COVID syndrome suffered from chronic fatigue at 6 months post-COVID-19 illness. Post-exertional symptom exacerbation affected most of the participants, and 58.7% met the scoring thresholds for people living with chronic fatigue syndrome/myalgic encephalomyelitis. These patients also had reduced capacity to work, be active and function both physically and socially. The impact of long COVID syndrome on health-related quality of life (HRQL) was substantial, despite the fact that the study sample consisted of younger patients, of whom almost half had no previous comorbidities.

Key Points

- Studies have examined more than 65 symptoms in patients with long COVID syndrome over 7 months post-acute infection.
- A variety of symptoms have been described in long COVID syndrome; long-term research is needed to study the associations between these symptoms and long COVID syndrome.
- Fatigue and post-exertional malaise are common manifestations in long COVID syndrome.

References

1. Davis HE, Assaf GS, McCorkell L, *et al.* Characterizing long COVID in an international cohort: 7 months of symptoms and their impact. *EClinicalMedicine* 2021; 38: 101019.
2. Twomey R, DeMars J, Franklin K, *et al.* Chronic fatigue and post-exertional malaise in people living with long COVID. Available from: https://doi.org/10.1101/2021.06.11.21258564.

Chapter 16

Differential diagnosis

Introduction

Long COVID syndrome should be investigated to rule out sinister causes before coming to a conclusive diagnosis. Positive test results for SARS-CoV-2 infection or a clinical picture of COVID-19 illness followed by characteristic persistent symptoms would point towards a diagnosis of long COVID syndrome, but only after ruling out sinister red flags and other causes that are amenable to treatment.

Ruling out other respiratory causes

Other respiratory causes have to be ruled out in patients who present with shortness of breath, cough and other respiratory symptoms. Apart from pulse oximetry, other useful investigations include chest X-ray, lung function testing and computed tomography of the chest.

Ruling out cardiac causes

The differential diagnosis of chest pain, palpitations, postural hypotension and arrhythmias includes cardiac causes unrelated to COVID-19. Therefore, it is vital to rule out acute cardiac conditions that can coexist with COVID-19.

Ruling out rheumatological causes

Chronic widespread pain and tiredness manifest similarly to fibromyalgia or chronic fatigue syndrome in patients with long COVID syndrome. Thus, it is very difficult to differentiate between 'primary' fibromyalgia and 'secondary' fibromyalgia as part of long COVID syndrome.

Ruling out neurological causes

The presence of delirium, hallucinations, muscle weakness, pain and neuropathic sensations requires specific relevant investigations to rule out neurological causes.

Ruling out endocrine causes

Endocrine, immunological and inflammatory causes should be considered as part of the differential diagnosis of symptoms of long COVID syndrome. It is therefore vital to rule out endocrine and related causes such as hypothyroidism or vitamin D/B_{12} deficiencies. Inflammatory conditions also should be excluded by appropriate blood tests.

Key Points

- It is vital to rule out sinister causes before reaching a diagnosis of long COVID syndrome.
- Positive testing for SARS-CoV-2 infection or a clinical picture of COVID-19 illness followed by typical symptoms of long COVID syndrome are required for a diagnosis of long COVID syndrome; however, other causes should also be excluded.

Chapter 17

Investigations in long COVID syndrome

Introduction

Long COVID syndrome can manifest with a range of over 200 symptoms, and it is vital to rule out sinister or treatable causes before reaching a diagnosis of the condition. Conducting appropriate investigations would help to reassure patients with long COVID syndrome, thereby helping them to engage better in their supported self-management rehabilitation pathway.

Confirmed or suspected COVID-19 illness

A diagnosis of long COVID syndrome requires that there is a history of new or ongoing symptoms for 4 weeks or more after the onset of confirmed or suspected COVID-19 illness. In people with no positive polymerase chain reaction (PCR) test, but with a clear history of COVID-19 illness followed by symptoms suggestive of long COVID syndrome, antigen or antibody tests should still be considered before making a diagnosis of long COVID syndrome.

Urgent referral in the presence of life-threatening symptoms

Patients should be urgently referred to acute hospital services if they present with emergency or life-threatening complications, including, but not limited to, the following:

- Severe hypoxaemia or desaturation on exercise.
- Severe signs of lung disease.
- Cardiac chest pain.
- Multisystem inflammatory syndrome in children.

Patient-tailored investigations

As symptoms and signs are varied in long COVID syndrome, investigations should be tailored to individual patients based on their presenting features. The goal is to rule out acute or life-threatening complications that can be either incidental (i.e. a new and unrelated diagnosis) or a consequence of COVID-19 illness.

If a different diagnosis not related to COVID-19 is suspected, appropriate investigations should be directed along that diagnostic line.

NICE guidelines on investigations

The National Institute for Health and Care Excellence (NICE) has published guidelines recommending routine blood tests to rule out inflammatory and other causes (■ Table 17.1). These tests can be easily offered to patients in primary care.

Table 17.1. Routine blood tests to rule out inflammatory and other causes.

Routine blood tests	What to look for?
Full blood count	Persistent inflammatory causes, white blood cell disorders (infection, lymphopenia, lymphocytosis) and signs of infection
	Anaemia and platelet disorders
C-reactive protein	Persistent inflammation if levels are high
Renal function tests (urea and electrolytes)	Renal disorders as sequelae of COVID-19, electrolyte abnormalities causing fatigue, muscle damage
Liver function tests	Liver damage, metabolic causes
Thyroid function tests	Causes of weakness/fatigue, other endocrine disorders
B-type natriuretic peptide	Heart failure
Ferritin	Inflammation, persistent thrombotic state
Creatine kinase	Muscle damage, inflammation

It may not be necessary to perform all tests listed above in all patients presenting with suspected long COVID syndrome-related symptoms. Investigations should be patient-specific and conducted based on patients' needs and presenting symptoms.

Exercise tolerance test

The 1-minute sit-to-stand test is a simple test to determine a person's exercise capacity. This test may not be suitable for patients with severe chest pain or extreme fatigue, and clinical judgement is vital to decide on patient suitability for taking the test.

A chair of standard height (46cm) without arm rests is positioned against a wall. The test is first demonstrated to the patient by the clinician. The patient is seated upright on the chair, with both knees and hips flexed at 90°, feet placed flat on the floor hip-width apart and arms rested with the hands on the thighs. The patient is asked to stand up from the chair and sit back down at self-paced speed, and to repeat this for 1 minute. The following test parameters are recorded: dyspnoea, fatigue, pulse oximetry and heart rate.

Tests for postural symptoms

For patients presenting with postural symptoms, including dizziness and palpitations, the autonomic nervous system should be tested. Heart rate and blood pressure measurements are taken in both supine and standing positions after 3 minutes (10 minutes if postural orthostatic tachycardia syndrome is suspected) and compared.

Chest X-ray

The British Thoracic Society guidelines recommend chest radiography for patients whose chest symptoms have not settled by 12 weeks post-hospital discharge. This should be accompanied by face-to-face clinical follow-up of the patient for evaluation of chest X-ray changes, as well as the patient's symptoms. Upon resolution of chest X-ray changes or if only minor, insignificant radiological changes (e.g. small areas of atelectasis) and the patient has made a good recovery, they should be discharged from care. If chest X-ray changes persist despite the patient clinically improving, further assessment is needed. The clinician must consider arranging additional chest X-ray imaging in 6–8 weeks to further evaluate the patient prior to potential discharge. However, it should be noted that chest X-ray alone might not be sufficient to rule out lung disease.

Further respiratory investigations

The British Thoracic Society guidelines recommend that if respiratory symptoms persist and abnormal chest X-ray findings have not resolved, then other tests should be considered, including:

- Pulmonary function tests.
- Echocardiography.
- Sputum microbiology.
- Investigations for pulmonary embolism or post-embolism complications.
- High-resolution computed tomography (CT) or CT pulmonary angiography.

Cardiovascular assessment

In the presence of cardiac symptoms, the clinician should consider troponin measurements to rule out acute coronary syndrome or myocarditis. D-dimer measurement may also be needed to exclude thromboembolic disease. However, these tests could be falsely positive in long COVID syndrome. Therefore, results should be correlated with the clinical picture to assess for the need for further tests.

Psychiatric assessment

It is important to assess for the risk of self-harm or suicide. Where required, urgent referral to the crisis team or the mental health team is vital.

Psychological assessment

Many patients with suspected or confirmed long COVID syndrome present with anxiety or other mood disorders, and will need referral to psychological services for assessment and treatment. Patients should be assessed for anxiety and depression, including with the use of evaluation questionnaires, depending on local expertise and availability.

Referral to specialist services

In the UK, in various parts of the country, the NHS has developed a number of integrated multidisciplinary services for patients with long COVID syndrome. Referral to these services should be considered for patients with persistent symptoms who have already undergone basic investigations. It is also vital to include assessments of quality of life when assessing patients with long COVID syndrome.

Key Points

- Long COVID syndrome can manifest with a range of over 200 symptoms and it is vital to rule out sinister or treatable causes.
- Investigations should be patient-specific and based on patients' presenting symptoms.
- Chest X-ray alone might not be sufficient to rule out lung disease.
- Psychiatric and/or psychological assessment is essential in long COVID syndrome to evaluate the effects of the condition on patients' quality of life.

References

1. National Institute for Health and Care Excellence (2020). COVID-19 rapid guideline: managing the long-term effects of COVID-19. NICE guideline [NG188]. Available from: https://www.nice.org.uk/guidance/ng188/chapter/Recommendations.

2. Ozalevli S, Ozden A, Itil O, *et al*. Comparison of the sit-to-stand test with 6 min walk test in patients with chronic obstructive pulmonary disease. *Respir Med* 2007; 101: 286–93.

3. British Thoracic Society (2020). British Thoracic Society guidance on respiratory follow-up of patients with a clinico-radiological diagnosis of COVID-19 pneumonia. Available from: https://www.brit-thoracic.org.uk/document-library/quality-improvement/covid-19/resp-follow-up-guidance-post-covid-pneumonia/.

4. Greenhalgh T, Knight M, A'Court C, *et al*. Management of post-acute covid-19 in primary care. *BMJ* 2020; 370: m3026.

Section III

Guidelines and policies

Chapter 18

NHS England plans for long COVID syndrome

Introduction

NHS England recognises that long COVID syndrome is a major problem and will represent a huge burden to health care services in the future. NHS England also recognises that long COVID syndrome is a multisystemic condition that is highly debilitating for many of its sufferers and is becoming increasingly widespread. Compared to many other countries, NHS England has been at the forefront in this pandemic by creating innovative pathways for the management of long COVID syndrome and implementing research in the condition.

Long COVID syndrome: NHS plan for 2021/2022

In June 2021, NHS England presented a key plan for 2021/2022, detailing a comprehensive strategy for the management of long COVID syndrome. This document covers the management for both ongoing symptomatic COVID-19 (5–12 weeks post-acute onset) and post-COVID-19 syndrome (12 weeks or more post-acute onset).

Five-point plan (October 2020)

As an initial response to the pandemic, NHS England set out a five-point plan in October 2020 that consisted of:

1. Advice for clinicians as well as patient information (guidelines published by the National Institute for Health and Care Excellence [NICE] in December 2020).
2. Establishing 89 assessment clinics in England for post-COVID syndrome.
3. Launching of the 'Your COVID recovery' website (providing specialist online rehabilitation support).
4. Allocating £50 million to the National Institute for Health Research to study long COVID syndrome.
5. Setting up the NHS Long COVID Taskforce (which includes participation from patients, clinicians and researchers).

Ten key steps from June 2021

In June 2021, NHS England updated its policy on the management of long COVID syndrome and provided further funding. The plans in this policy included:

1. Allocating £70 million to expand support services to tackle long COVID syndrome (with £24 million already spent on clinic set-up).
2. Allocating £30 million for primary care support to enhance general practice services and support relevant education and training.
3. Ensuring care coordination for joined-up and priority-based clinical needs.
4. Setting up 15 post-COVID syndrome assessment hubs for children and young people.
5. Provision of standard rehabilitation pathway packages.
6. Extending the use of the 'Your COVID Recovery' online platform for rehabilitation.
7. Data collection and publication.
8. Ensuring equity of access, outcomes and experience.
9. Creating a national learning network to promote good clinical practice.
10. Supporting NHS staff suffering from long COVID syndrome.

NHS England has proposed that additional funding will be allocated to integrated care systems (ICS) to ensure that financial support goes to the right services for diagnostics, treatment and rehabilitation. There is particular emphasis on services adopting a multidisciplinary approach, including physical, cognitive, psychological and psychiatric assessments, with the aim to provide consistent services and face-to-face appointments when appropriate. This proposal ensures that patients who have never been admitted to hospital due to COVID-19 illness or who have never tested positive for COVID-19 are also included in this care pathway.

Care pathways and resource projection for patients with long COVID syndrome

Early estimates of resources have been projected for three different pathways as follows (■ Figure 18.1):

- Tier 1: 30–50% of patients needing supported self-management.
- Tier 2: 18–30% of patients treated in primary care or the community.
- Tier 3: 20–50% needing specialist services and rehabilitation pathways.

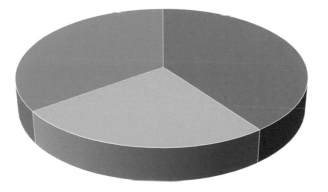

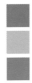

Tier 1: Self-manage 30-50%

Tier 2: Community support 18-30%

Tier 3: Specialist support 20-50%

Figure 18.1. Pathways of rehabilitation in long COVID syndrome.

Three core principles are embedded in these care pathways, including:

- Personalised care.
- A multidisciplinary approach to rehabilitation.
- Supporting and enabling self-care.

NHS Long COVID Taskforce

Given the urgent need for information on long COVID syndrome, NHS England has focused its efforts on ensuring clarity when creating referral pathways to remove barriers to access long COVID services and maximise efficiency in service provision. General practitioners and other health care professionals need the correct and relevant information in a timely manner, as well as good communication channels, so they can help patients receive appropriate investigations and treatment — safely and consistently. In November 2020, NHS England launched a new taskforce to tackle long COVID syndrome, including patients, charities, researchers and clinicians. The aim is to produce information and support materials to educate and prepare patients and clinicians, so they can develop a better understanding of the condition.

Key Points

- For management of long COVID syndrome, the NHS produced a five-point plan in October 2020, followed by a comprehensive ten-point plan in June 2021.
- A total of 89 long COVID assessment specialist clinics and 15 assessment hubs for children have been set up by the NHS.
- A budget of more than £100 million has been allocated by the NHS to the management of long COVID syndrome in the UK (as of June 2021).

References

1.   NHS England and NHS Improvement (2021). Long COVID: the NHS plan for 2021/22. Version 1, June 2021. Available from: https://www.england.nhs.uk/coronavirus/wp-content/uploads/sites/52/2021/06 /C1312-long-covid-plan-june-2021.pdf.

2.   Patient Safety Learning (2021). Long Covid patient experience: NHS England Taskforce on Long Covid (4 February 2021). Available from: https://www.pslhub.org/learn/coronavirus-covid19/patient-recovery/long-covid-patient-experience-nhs-england-taskforce-on-long-covid-4-february-2021-r4209/.

Chapter 19

NICE guidelines on long COVID syndrome

Introduction

The National Institute for Health and Care Excellence (NICE) is an organisation in the UK that provides evidence-based guidance and advice to improve health and social care. This forms the basis of the health care commissioners' decision-making process to allocate resources to services according to needs in health and social care.

Given the magnitude of the challenges of long COVID syndrome, NICE (jointly with the Royal College of General Practitioners and the Scottish Intercollegiate Guidelines Network) published, in December 2020, a rapid guideline for the management of long-term effects of COVID-19. The guideline covers the definition for the condition and guidance on assessment, investigations, management and service organisation.

NICE criteria for long COVID syndrome

NICE guidelines have clarified the criteria for the definition of long COVID syndrome very succintly; it clearly differentiates four different conditions as below (see ■ Figure 19.1):

- Acute COVID-19: signs and symptoms of COVID-19 for up to 4 weeks.
- Ongoing symptomatic COVID-19: signs and symptoms of COVID-19 from 4 to 12 weeks.

- Post-COVID-19 syndrome: signs and symptoms that develop during or after an infection consistent with COVID-19 and continue for more than 12 weeks.
- Long COVID syndrome: signs and symptoms present from 4 weeks onwards, including both ongoing symptomatic COVID-19 and post-COVID-19 syndrome.

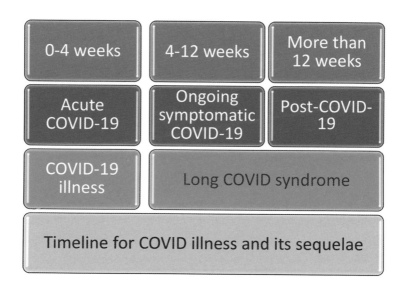

Figure 19.1. Time course for COVID-19.

The NICE guidelines provide clear advice with regard to identifying and managing patients with long COVID syndrome as outlined below.

Identifying people with long COVID syndrome

- Symptoms persisting after a suspected or confirmed COVID-19 diagnosis.

- Information provided in accessible formats that can be easily understood.
- Initial consultation given if symptoms persist for 4 weeks or more after acute COVID-19 illness.
- Screening questionnaire to be considered as part of the initial consultation.
- Any hospital-discharged patients to be followed up after 6 weeks via video or telephone consultation.

Assessment

- A holistic, patient-centred approach.
- Comprehensive clinical history taking; examination to assess for physical, cognitive and psychological/psychiatric symptoms, as well as functional abilities.
- Use of a validated screening tool for cognitive symptoms.

Investigations and referral

- Urgent referral to acute services if any signs or symptoms of acute or life-threatening complications, including, but not limited to:
  - severe hypoxaemia or desaturation on exercise;
  - severe lung disease;
  - cardiac chest pain;
  - multisystem inflammatory syndrome in children.
- Investigations tailored to the patient's signs and symptoms, and ruling out acute or life-threatening complications.
- Blood tests: full blood count, renal and liver function tests, C-reactive protein, ferritin, B-type natriuretic peptide and thyroid function tests.
- To perform the 1-minute sit-to-stand test for an exercise tolerance assessment; appropriate tests if postural symptoms present (see Chapter 17).
- Chest X-ray if continuing respiratory symptoms after 12 weeks post-acute onset.
- Psychiatric and psychological assessments.

Care planning

- Self-management advised.
- Referral to integrated multidisciplinary assessment services if needed.
- Referral to specialist care for specific complications.

Management

- Self-management, as well as supported self-management.
- Multidisciplinary rehabilitation, including physical, psychological and psychiatric.
- Personalised rehabilitation and management plan.

Follow-up and monitoring

- To agree plans with the patient, based on shared decision-making, tailored to the patient's needs.
- To continue supported self-monitoring, as well as patient education.

For the full guidance, see 'References'.

The NICE guideline emphasises information sharing and continuity of care and gives advice on specific service organisation. It concludes by highlighting the need for prioritising research on the underlying pathophysiology of long COVID syndrome as an urgent focus, with particular emphasis on characterising clusters of symptoms (phenotypes), risk factors, prognostic markers and defining the trajectory of long COVID syndrome.

The NICE guideline also covers the need for interventions in specific patient groups with mental health conditions and learning difficulties and those with specific cultural and language barriers.

Controversies in the NICE guideline

The ME Association has voiced its concerns on the use of graded exercise recommended by NICE. There have also been concerns by some health organisations on the use of cognitive behavioural therapy, quoting its ineffectiveness in long COVID syndrome. NICE has advised caution when using graded exercise in those suffering from severe symptoms of long COVID syndrome and has planned for a future update on its recommendations.

Key Points

- NICE published its guideline on long COVID syndrome in December 2020, recognising the huge burden of this condition on the health care system in providing patient care.
- The NICE guideline defines long COVID syndrome as a condition that includes both ongoing symptomatic COVID-19 and post-COVID-19 syndrome in symptomatic patients after 4 weeks of infection.
- NICE stresses that if a patient has a suspected history or features of COVID-19 and presents with symptoms of long COVID syndrome after 4 weeks, they should be considered for further assessment and appropriate management, even if they do not have a confirmatory test for COVID-19.
- The NICE guideline emphasises a holistic, patient-centred approach, with supported self-management as the main goal.

References

1.   National Institute for Health and Care Excellence (2020). COVID-19 rapid guideline: managing the long-term effects of COVID-19. NICE guideline [NG188]. Available from: https://www.nice.org.uk/guidance/ng188.

Chapter 20

ME Association guidelines on long COVID syndrome

Introduction

The ME (myalgic encephalomyelitis) Association has been supporting people who suffer from post-viral fatigue syndromes for many years. In the context of COVID-19, it was becoming clear that many people were not improving after their acute illness, even after several weeks. The ME Association was one of the first to publish management and guidance protocols on post-viral fatigue syndrome in April 2020, which were updated in November 2020 and again in April 2021.

The ME Association noted that almost all sufferers of long COVID syndrome have been self-managed at home, with the majority experiencing debilitating fatigue, with or without lung or heart symptoms. According to the Office for National Statistics, one in five people (equating to one million people) in the UK remain symptomatic at 5 weeks after the initial COVID-19 illness. One in seven are symptomatic at 12 weeks post-acute illness, and around 70,000 people are still symptomatic after 1 year. One in five sufferers experience a significant impact of their symptoms on their day-to-day activities.

Further, according to the University of Leicester/PHOSP-COVID study, seven in ten patients admitted to hospital with COVID-19 still have not recovered at 5 months post-discharge. One in four patients have significant anxiety or depression.

Key messages from the ME Association on long COVID syndrome

The ME Association has published the following key guidance on long COVID syndrome:

- There is a significant female preponderance; many people with long COVID syndrome are fit, young adults (aged 20–50 years).
- Patients with long COVID syndrome who develop serious complications are commonly male and aged over 50 years.
- Fatigue is the most debilitating symptom.
- Some have respiratory, heart or other symptoms similar to those present in acute infection.
- Although there is no specific drug treatment for long COVID syndrome, management focuses on improving sufferers' activity and energy levels.
- A more flexible approach is needed in those patients needing cardiorespiratory rehabilitation.
- The outlook for people with long COVID syndrome is uncertain.
- Some patients with long COVID syndrome are steadily improving; however, many remain unwell and become chronically ill, with fluctuating symptom severity.

Long COVID syndrome and myalgic encephalomyelitis/ chronic fatigue syndrome

According to the ME Association, people who already suffer from myalgic encephalomyelitis (ME) or chronic fatigue syndrome (CFS) may have significant exacerbation or relapse of their ME/CFS symptoms in long COVID syndrome.

Patient self-reporting on long COVID syndrome

The ME Association has provided further clear-cut guidelines to take the symptoms of long COVID syndrome seriously as below:

- The ME Association recommends that patients need to be listened to and their concerns acknowledged — reports of their symptoms should not be dismissed as symptoms of anxiety or depression just because of a lack of blood test evidence or objective evidence.

- General practitioners should provide ongoing support, rather than giving a diagnosis with no further interventions.
- Specialist referral might be needed for further assessment and investigation if there are significant symptoms.
- A multidisciplinary approach is essential for the management of patients in both primary and secondary care.

Red flag symptoms

The ME Association lists the following as red flag symptoms:

- Continuing fever or periodic spikes.
- Persistent cough, shortness of breath or other respiratory symptoms.
- Chest pain or palpitations.
- Weight loss.
- Feeling anxious or depressed.
- Persistent diarrhoea or abdominal pain.

Management guidelines from the ME Association

The ME Association has recommended the following management plans for long COVID syndrome:

- Convalescence: rest, relaxation and cautiously increasing activity levels.
- Four important basic management principles, including:
  - planning: spreading physical and mental activities thoughout the day;
  - prioritising: lower priority activities can be deferred or omitted;
  - delegating: delegating activities or tasks to family or friends if possible;
  - explaining: explaining about the condition to employers and work colleagues, family and social contacts.
- Activity and energy management: pacing.
- Sleep management.
- Managing neurological symptoms, cognitive problems, orthostatic problems and pain.
- Drug treatments for symptomatic relief.
- Managing mental well-being and relationships.

- Good nutrition and fluid intake.
- Managing education and employment.
- Dealing with financial difficulties.

Prognosis of long COVID syndrome

According to the ME Association, the outlook for people with long COVID syndrome is highly uncertain, given the limited current knowledge on the condition.

Concerning recommendations from the National Institute for Health and Care Excellence (NICE) on the management of long COVID syndrome, the ME Association is not in favour of cognitive behavioural therapy or graded exercise therapy. However, further research is needed and future updates might change the recommendations based on emerging evidence.

Key Points

- The ME Association has produced guidelines on long COVID syndrome, with regular updates based on emerging evidence.
- Fatigue is the most debilitating symptom in long COVID syndrome.
- Although there is no specific drug treatment for long COVID syndrome, management should focus on improving sufferers' activity and energy levels.

References

1. Shepherd C, for the ME Association (2021). Long COVID and ME/CFS. Available from: https://meassociation.org.uk/wp-content/uploads/Long-covid-and-MECFS-April-2021.pdf.

Chapter 21

American guidelines for long COVID syndrome

Introduction

In the United States, given the magnitude of the effects of long COVID syndrome, the White House has announced that millions of Americans who suffer from long-term sequelae of COVID-19 illness should not face higher premiums or refusal of health insurance because of this new condition.

The Centers for Disease Control and Prevention (CDC) has issued clear guidelines on the long-term effects of COVID-19, along with interim guidance on how to assess and care for patients with long COVID syndrome.

CDC guidance on long COVID syndrome

The CDC is clear that post-COVID illness encompasses a wide range of new, returning or ongoing health problems that people experience four or more weeks after their initial infection with SARS-CoV-2.

Interim guidance on post-COVID conditions

The CDC has provided interim guidance on the management of post-COVID conditions as below:

- Many patients can be managed by primary care providers, with a patient-centred approach aiming to optimise patients' quality of life and function.
- Objective laboratory or imaging findings should not be used as the only measure of a patient's well-being. Lack of abnormal findings does not invalidate the existence, severity or importance of a patient's symptoms or condition.
- Shared decision-making, along with setting achievable goals, is needed.
- The approach to treatment should focus on specific symptoms or conditions.
- A comprehensive management plan should aim to improve physical, mental and social well-being.

The guidance from the CDC is likely to change over time, as new evidence on post-COVID conditions emerges.

National Institutes of Health guidelines on long COVID syndrome

Given there are no specific treatments for the persistent effects of COVID-19 illness, with no case definition or specific time frame for long COVID syndrome, the National Institutes of Health (NIH) has recommended strategies focusing on general management.

Other recommendations from the NIH include further research and rigorous observational cohort studies to understand the pathophysiology of post-acute COVID-19 sequelae, as well as the clinical course of the condition, and identifying management strategies for affected patients.

Key Points

- The CDC has issued clear guidelines on the long-term effects of COVID-19 illness, along with interim guidance on how to assess and care for affected patients.
- Guidance from the CDC will be updated regularly as new evidence emerges.
- The NIH has recommended for further research and rigorous observational cohort studies on long COVID syndrome.

References

1. The White House. COVID-19: The Biden–Harris plan to beat COVID-19. Available from: https://www.whitehouse.gov/priorities/covid-19/.
2. Centers for Disease Control and Prevention (2021). Post-COVID conditions. Available from: https://www.cdc.gov/coronavirus/2019-ncov/long-term-effects.html.
3. Centers for Disease Control and Prevention (2021). Evaluating and caring for patients with post-COVID conditions: interim guidance. Available from: https://www.cdc.gov/coronavirus/2019-ncov/hcp/clinical-care/post-covid-index.html.
4. National Institutes of Health (2021). Clinical spectrum of SARS-CoV-2 infection. Available from: https://www.covid19treatmentguidelines.nih.gov/overview/clinical-spectrum/.

Chapter 22

Guidelines from other health organisations

Introduction

As data on long COVID syndrome have just been emerging, more evidence-based information is yet to be available. Meanwhile, many countries and health organisations have adopted a cautious and precautionary approach, recommending a comprehensive management plan to deal with the huge impact of long COVID syndrome on society as a whole.

Guidance from the World Health Organization (Europe)

In May 2020, the World Health Organization (WHO) Regional Office for Europe produced a technical working guidance for strengthening the health system response to the COVID-19 pandemic across long-term care services. The guidance emphasises the need to prioritise maintenance of long-term care services during the COVID-19 pandemic through an effective governance mechanism.

Guidance from the Scottish Intercollegiate Guidelines Network on long COVID syndrome

The Scottish Intercollegiate Guidelines Network (SIGN), as part of Healthcare Improvement Scotland, has published a patient booklet on long

COVID syndrome, jointly with the National Institute for Health and Care Excellence (NICE) and Royal College of General Practitioners (RCGP).

Guidance from the European Agency for Safety and Health at Work

The European Agency for Safety and Health at Work (EU-OSHA) has produced two sets of guidance on the challenges faced by returning workers after COVID-19 illness and long COVID syndrome.

EU-OSHA guidance to workers

- This guidance states that returning to work after long COVID syndrome can be 'tough'.
- Although affected patients might be struggling with their daily activities, they might feel compelled to work for financial reasons or for social reasons to support their mental health.
- Although recovery can be slow, many people improve with time; as we gain a better understanding of the condition, progress in finding appropriate treatments should be expected.
- Return to work is part of the recovery process; however, this should initially be phased and flexible.
- It is sensible for workers and employers to work together towards a return to work that is most productive for all concerned.
- Long COVID syndrome can have unusual patterns — relapses as well as phases with sometimes new and bizarre symptoms.
- Return to work adjustments should be tailored to the affected worker, depending on their health problems, their ability to function and their job role.

EU-OSHA guidance to managers

- EU-OSHA has produced a guide for managers in this context, highlighting that line managers have a significant influence on a successful return to work of their staff; what they do and how they behave can affect the returning worker's ability to return to work and to remain in work.

- Managers do not need to be an expert in long COVID syndrome but should be able to support the returning worker, listen to their concerns and act where they can.
- Five key steps for the manager in supporting the returning worker include:
  - staying in touch while the worker is absent from work;
  - preparing for the worker's return to work;
  - having a return-to-work conversation;
  - providing support in the early stages after return to work;
  - providing ongoing support, as well as regular reviews.
- Occupational health services can provide support by effectively carrying out appropriate workplace risk assessments for an optimal return to work tailored to the needs of the returning worker who suffers, or has suffered, from long COVID syndrome.

Health systems and policy analysis guidance from the World Health Organization

The WHO Regional Office for Europe has published a health systems and policy analysis guidance, entitled 'In the wake of the pandemic', to help prepare for long COVID syndrome. Many people struggle to recover from acute COVID-19 illness and often suffer from disabling symptoms that last for weeks or months, resulting in long-lasting disabilities in some cases. Of note, the guidance foreword ends with an alarming statement: 'The legacy of COVID-19 will, sadly, be with us for a long time'. Key points of the guidance are summarised below:

- Long COVID syndrome has a serious impact on people's ability to go back to work or have a social life; it affects their mental health.
- It has significant economic consequences for patients, their families and society as a whole.
- There is a need for multidisciplinary and multispecialty approaches to patient assessment and management.
- New care pathways and contextually appropriate guidelines should be developed in collaboration with patients and their families.
- Wider implications include consideration of employment rights, sick pay policies and access to benefit and disability benefit packages.

- Patients should be involved in fostering self-care and self-help, as well as in raising awareness of long COVID syndrome and the service/research needs that it generates.

Key Points

- The WHO Regional Office for Europe has highlighted the need to strengthen long-term care services during the COVID pandemic.
- SIGN has produced a patient booklet on long COVID syndrome.
- EU-OSHA has published guidance for workers and managers on how to deal with the effects of long COVID syndrome.
- WHO health systems and policy analysis guidance has emphasised the need for multidisciplinary and multispecialty approaches to tackle long COVID syndrome.

References

1. World Health Organization Regional Office for Europe (2020). Strengthening the health system response to COVID-19: preventing and managing the COVID-19 pandemic across long-term care services in the WHO European Region. Technical Working Guidance #6. Available from: https://apps.who.int/iris/bitstream/handle/10665/333067/WHO-EURO-2020-804-40539-54460-eng.pdf?sequence=1&isAllowed=y.

2. Scottish Intercollegiate Guidelines Network (2020). Long COVID: a booklet for people who have signs and symptoms that continue or develop after acute COVID-19. Available from: https://www.sign.ac.uk/media/1825/sign-long-covid-patient-booklet-v2.pdf.

3. European Agency for Safety and Health at Work (2021). COVID-19 infection and long COVID: guide for workers. Available from: https://osha.europa.eu/en/publications/covid-19-infection-and-long-covid-guide-workers/view.

4. European Agency for Safety and Health at Work (2021). COVID-19 infection and long COVID: guide for managers. Available from: https://osha.europa.eu/en/publications/covid-19-infection-and-long-covid-guide-managers/view.

5. World Health Organization Regional Office for Europe (2021). In the wake of the pandemic: preparing for long COVID. Policy brief 39. Health Systems and Policy Analysis. Available from: https://apps.who.int/iris/bitstream/handle/10665/339629/Policy-brief-39-1997-8073-eng.pdf.

Section IV

Management of long COVID syndrome

Chapter 23

Management principles for long COVID syndrome

Introduction

The evidence base for strategies used to manage the relatively new condition of long COVID syndrome is limited. New research is continuously emerging, with many studies focusing on developing strategies to improve the quality of life of sufferers of long COVID syndrome. This chapter will deal with the general principles of management of long COVID syndrome, with subsequent chapters covering specific management in detail.

Course of recovery

Approximately 10% of people with COVID-19 experience prolonged illness. Many patients recover immediately post-acute infection, albeit slowly, with holistic support, rest and symptomatic treatment, and show gradual improvement in functional activity. Some patients might need a longer recovery period, while others may suffer from significant deterioration in their quality of life.

Self-management

Guidelines from the National Institute for Health and Care Excellence (NICE) recommend self-management, as well as supported self-management, as the main strategies in the management of long COVID syndrome.

Patient-specific management plan

Long COVID syndrome is a multisystem condition that requires a whole-patient management approach aiming to improve functional status. However, knowledge of this condition is still evolving and will continue to improve with future studies.

Lifestyle changes should be recommended, as this is a window of opportunity to advise patients on the importance of taking appropriate rest, proper nutrition/healthy diet, hydration, sleep hygiene, reducing alcohol intake and smoking cessation — all of which are standard recommendations given to patients recovering from any illness, to promote physical and mental well-being.

Shared decision-making with the patient is important, especially when planning for appropriate support and rehabilitation. The management plan should be agreed upon with the patient, while giving specific advice on self-management.

Exclusion of serious complications

It is vital to exclude serious ongoing complications or comorbidities. At the same time, it is important to manage the patient pragmatically and symptomatically, with the emphasis on holistic support, while avoiding unnecessary over-investigations.

Cardiorespiratory complications, commonly seen in long COVID syndrome, should be recognised and treated, and affected patients referred to an appropriate acute care pathway.

Pacing of patient recovery

Recovery from long COVID syndrome is often slow and gradual. Improvement in energy levels and shortness of breath can take a protracted course. Careful pacing of recovery, prioritisation and modest goal setting are vital when managing patients with long COVID syndrome.

Mental health

Anxiety and depression are seen in long COVID syndrome, which are further exacerbated by social isolation and loneliness. Sleep problems should be assessed for and managed. A minority of patients will need referral to mental health services. However, it is important to assess all patients with long COVID syndrome and to educate them on simple strategies to improve their mood, sleep and quality of life.

Referral to specialist rehabilitation services

Many patients with long COVID syndrome go through a slow and gradual recovery phase. However, some might need referral to specialist rehabilitation services.

Any rehabilitation services should take into account patients' comorbidities that could affect their recovery progress or their ability to take part in rehabilitation programmes.

Pulmonary rehabilitation

Patients with long COVID syndrome who show significant respiratory symptoms will need referral for pulmonary rehabilitation. Pulmonary rehabilitation programmes should focus on personalised evaluation and treatment, including education, behavioural modification and graded exercise training. However, patients with fatigue as their predominant problem need a different or modified pathway.

Management of fatigue

Rehabilitation experts in long COVID syndrome have found that profound fatigue is the main barrier to recovery. All interventions in this regard are based on indirect evidence, extrapolated from chronic fatigue syndrome and other medical conditions. The role of graded exercise in chronic fatigue syndrome associated with long COVID syndrome, as recommended by NICE, has proved controversial, with strong objections to these guideline recommendations (see Chapter 19) from some patient groups. If a patient has significant shortness of breath or severe fatigue or muscle aches, or if a patient has other constitutional symptoms such as fever or cough, it might not be advisable to suggest graded exercise or behavioural modifications at that time. Patient-specific and individualised plans, with full participation of the patient, are vital in the management of long COVID-related fatigue. Good understanding, as well as providing explanations, support and reassurance, from the clinician goes a long way in the management of these patients.

Exercise rehabilitation recommendations

The Stanford Hall consensus statement for exercise rehabilitation in long COVID syndrome describes the following recommendations for patients recovering from COVID-19 illness (all with a level of evidence 5, which is the highest level of evidence):

- Asymptomatic contacts: to continue exercises as per normal exercise level.
- Very mild symptoms — may or may not be due to COVID-19: to limit to light activity (≤3 metabolic equivalent of tasks [METs]), but also to limit the number of sedentary periods; to increase rest periods if symptoms deteriorate.
- Mild/moderate COVID-19 illness: to trial 1 week of low-level stretching and light muscle-strengthening activity before cardiovascular sessions.
- COVID-19 with severe symptoms: to avoid exercise (>3 METs or equivalent) for 2–3 weeks after cessation of symptoms.

- Patients who required oxygen therapy or had lymphopenia: to assess for radiological pulmonary changes and to perform pulmonary function tests; a gradual increase in exercise should be based on symptoms.
- Patients with cardiac problems: to commence a specific cardiac rehabilitation programme tailored to the patient's impairment and needs.
- Patients who had myocarditis and have a physically demanding job: to take complete rest for 3–6 months.

Pathways

Most patients with long COVID syndrome recover symptomatically with time, while supported in primary care. For those patients who remain symptomatic, NICE recommends three management pathways:

- Some patients will need integrated and coordinated management from primary care and rehabilitation and mental health services.
- Some will need referral to an integrated multidisciplinary assessment service.
- Some will need referral to specialist care for specific complications.

It is important to follow up these patients, to monitor their overall symptomatic trajectory. Symptoms can fluctuate and recur, such that patients may require different levels of support at different times.

Encouraging patients to 'own' their recovery

Self-management and supported self-management are the key for recovery once red flag conditions have been ruled out. The 'three Ps' principle (Pace, Plan, Prioritise) provides a framework that will facilitate structured discussions between clinicians and patients on their rehabilitation from long COVID syndrome.

Key Points

- Self-management and supported self-management are the key to recovery, once red flag symptoms have been ruled out.
- Recovery from long COVID syndrome can be slow and gradual; a patient-specific management plan should be made, with proper discussion and agreement with the patient.
- Exercise rehabilitation programmes can vary, depending on the patient's symptoms.

References

1. Greenhalgh T, Knight M, A'Court C, *et al*. Management of post-acute COVID-19 in primary care. *BMJ* 2020; 370: m3026.

2. Crook H, Raza S, Nowell J, *et al*. Long COVID — mechanisms, risk factors, and management. *BMJ* 2021; 374: n1648.

3. National Institute for Health and Care Excellence (2020). COVID-19 rapid guideline: managing the long-term effects of COVID-19. NICE guideline [NG188]. Available from: https://www.nice.org.uk/guidance/ng188.

4. Chaudhry A, Master H (2020). Top tips: managing long COVID. Guidelines in practice. Available from: https://www.guidelinesinpractice.co.uk/infection/top-tips-managing-long-covid/455742.article.

5. Barker-Davies RM, O'Sullivan O, Senaratne KPP, *et al*. The Stanford Hall consensus statement for post-COVID-19 rehabilitation. Consensus statement. *Br J Sports Med* 2020; 54: 949–59.

Chapter 24

Long COVID assessment centres

Introduction

Given the scale of the problem of long COVID syndrome affecting England, NHS England has set up specialist assessment centres for assessment and rehabilitation of patients symptomatic of long COVID syndrome. These centres have been undergoing huge development, while increasing in numbers across the country.

Initial start of assessment centres

In October 2020, NHS England and NHS Improvement announced a five-point plan to support patients with long COVID syndrome (see Chapter 18). As part of this plan, £10 million funding was invested in setting up specialist long COVID assessment centres across England.

In December 2020, NHS England announced the opening of 69 specialist long COVID assessment clinics across the country. The aim is to bring together doctors, nurses, physiotherapists and occupational therapists, so they can provide both physical and psychological assessments, as well as appropriate treatment and rehabilitation services, to referred patients with long COVID syndrome. At around the same time, the National Institute for Health and Care Excellence (NICE) published guidance on best practice for recognising, investigating and rehabilitating patients with long COVID syndrome. Patients can be referred to these specialist assessment centres by their general practitioner or other health care professionals, only when other possible underlying causes for symptoms have been ruled out first.

NHS England has also launched a Long COVID Taskforce, with the involvement of patients, charities, researchers and clinicians, to produce support materials for clinicians and patients.

Expansion of specialist services to include children and young people

In June 2021, NHS England launched specialist long COVID clinics for children and young people, as part of a £100 million expansion of the five-point plan. This initiative comprised the opening of 15 paediatric hubs. Estimations showed that 7.4% of children aged 2–11 years and 8.2% of those aged 12–16 years have reported continued symptoms of long COVID syndrome.

This service expansion also included £30 million allocated to general practitioners to improve the diagnosis and care of patients with long COVID syndrome, as well as to improve online patient support services ('Your COVID Recovery' website — https://www.yourcovidrecovery.nhs.uk/). According to NHS England, this plan aims to deal with the COVID 'legacy', which clearly demonstrates the seriousness of the problem of long COVID syndrome that needs tackling with long-term plans from the NHS.

By July 2021, NHS England had already spent £34 million on developing specialist long COVID assessment clinics. The government has since pledged an extra £70 million to expand these services and develop paediatric hubs, some of which will also go towards integrated care systems (ICS) to ensure provision of the right services for diagnostics, treatment and rehabilitation in community, acute, tertiary and mental health settings.

Long COVID: the NHS plan for 2021/22

With currently 89 specialist long COVID assessment clinics across England, it is estimated that these clinics will receive over 1500 referrals per week. There were over 1.5 million visits to the 'Your COVID Recovery' website in just a few months, and over 100 rehabilitation services have been trained to support patients in using specialist online rehabilitation support platform.

NHS England announced a long COVID registry for patients attending long COVID assessment clinics which was established in July 2021. This registry will help to understand the patient journey, as well as support clinical, operational and research activities, by linking data gathered across the country. The aim of the registry is to provide an understanding of patient access to these clinics based on health inequalities.

NHS England also asked for all ICS to provide by mid-July 2021 fully staffed long COVID service plans to regional teams that cover the whole pathway from primary to specialist care, including for children. These plans should show how they meet the commissioning guidance for the management of patients with long COVID syndrome and maximise the use of the online rehabilitation platform for supported patient self-management.

Commissioning for long COVID assessment clinics

In April 2021, NHS England published commissioning guidance for long COVID assessment clinics. The setting for this service is determined locally and may be primary care-, secondary care- or community-based, as long as there is prompt access to appropriate diagnostics and treatments. The service should ensure coverage of the population in each setting.

The commissioning guidance recommends referral of patients with long COVID syndrome presenting with (but not limited to) the following:

- Severe hypoxaemia or oxygen desaturation on exercise.
- Signs of severe lung disease.
- Cardiac chest pain.
- Multisystem inflammatory syndrome (in children).

The commissioning guidance quotes three principles of care for long COVID syndrome:

- Personalised care.
- Multidisciplinary support and rehabilitation.
- Supporting and enabling self-care.

The guidance also gives details of the service design, workforce needed, pathways, data and management information and measurement outcomes.

Core features of long COVID support services

- Services must be multidisciplinary and offer physical, cognitive, psychological and psychiatric assessments.
- Services must make provision for all those affected, including those who have never been admitted to hospital or tested for COVID-19.
- Services must ensure equity of access.

Modelling demand for specialist services

Many individuals with long COVID syndrome might not seek NHS help. Of those who seek help, many can be supported by the primary care or community team. Few will need specialist assessment. NHS England has estimated that around 2.9% of people who have been affected by COVID-19 illness will go on to need NHS support for long-term symptoms — including around 342,000 people as of June 2021 — and these numbers are likely to increase over time. Of these patients, 20% to 50% are classified as Tier 3 patients (see Chapter 18) who will need support from specialist assessment clinics and rehabilitation programmes.

Key Points

- The NHS has invested £100 million in the development of specialist long COVID assessment clinics across England to aid in patient rehabilitation and recovery.
- The comprehensive 'Long COVID: the NHS plan for 2021/22' provides guidance in service provision to support recovery of patients suffering from long COVID syndrome.
- In April 2021, the NHS released streamlined commissioning guidance for specialist long COVID assessment clinics.
- Nearly 3% of those who have been affected by COVID-19 illness will need NHS support for long-term symptoms; of these, an estimated 20–50% will require specialist assessment services.

References

1. NHS England and NHS Improvement (2020). Post-COVID syndrome (long COVID). Available from: https://www.england.nhs.uk/coronavirus/post-covid-syndrome-long-covid/.

2. NHS England (2020). Long COVID patients to get help at more than 60 clinics. Available from: https://www.england.nhs.uk/2020/12/long-covid-patients-to-get-help-at-more-than-60-clinics/.

3. NHS England (2021). NHS sets up specialist young people's services in £100 million long COVID care expansion. Available from: https://www.england.nhs.uk/2021/06/nhs-sets-up-specialist-young-peoples-services-in-100-million-long-covid-care-expansion/.

4. NHS England (2021). National guidance for post-COVID syndrome assessment clinics. Version 2, 26 April 2021. Available from: https://www.england.nhs.uk/coronavirus/wp-content/uploads/sites/52/2020/11/C1248-national-guidance-post-covid-syndrome-assessment-clinics-v2.pdf.

5. NHS England (2021). Long COVID: the NHS plan for 2021/22. Version 1, June 2021. Available from: https://www.england.nhs.uk/coronavirus/wp-content/uploads/sites/52/2021/06/C1312-long-covid-plan-june-2021.pdf.

Chapter 25

Online recovery and rehabilitation platforms

Introduction

In this era of modern technology, it would be quite inconceivable not to include the creation of online platforms when planning and designing management pathways for patient recovery and rehabilitation. This is particularly relevant in these times of lockdown and social restrictions. It is thus vital to harness the technological capabilities at our disposal to support patients with long COVID syndrome in their recovery.

'Your COVID Recovery' online support

In October 2020, NHS England and NHS Improvement announced a five-point plan for long COVID support, which included the introduction of the second phase of the 'Your COVID Recovery' online platform. Details of expansion of the platform were released in June 2021 as part of the 'Long COVID: the NHS plan for 2021/22' — https://www.yourcovidrecovery.nhs.uk/. The ten-point plan stresses on extending the use of the 'Your COVID Recovery' online rehabilitation platform, requiring local NHS systems to 'ramp up' the online support for patient self-management by mid-July 2021. The aim is to enable online content translation into more than 100 languages through improved functionality, as well as ensuring improved accessibility by including easy-read options and a printed manual which replicates online content.

Online self-management digital tool

As long COVID syndrome is a long-term condition, supported self-care is an important part of management where clinically appropriate. Online platforms can help in this context by helping to generate data and information that could be collated for research on pathways and efficacy of interventions.

It is estimated that 10% of patients in the UK with long COVID syndrome will receive supervised treatment via the 'Your COVID Recovery' online platform, and another 10% will self-manage using digital app support. It is estimated that 20% of long COVID syndrome patients seen in clinics in the UK will be followed up via digital rehabilitation platforms.

Features of 'Your COVID Recovery' platform

'Your COVID Recovery' is a website providing support, information and advice, with over 1.5 million site visits over just a few months since its launch. The online support helps to manage, and thereby alleviate, the physical and psychological impact of long COVID syndrome on the day-to-day living of sufferers.

It also provides a personalised and tailored module package under a clinician's supervision. It enables individualised goal setting, and resources can be selected accordingly to help achieve treatment goals.

The website is being expanded to allow patient self-referral.

Practicalities of 'Your COVID Recovery' platform

Patients with persistent symptoms of long COVID syndrome will have face-to-face consultations with their local multidisciplinary rehabilitation team. Following this, they will be offered a personalised package of online-based care for a duration of 12 weeks that includes:

- A personalised package based on symptoms and what is important to the patient.
- Access to the local clinical team who can respond to enquiries from the patient.
- Online peer support, particularly helpful to those recovering alone at home.
- An exercise programme for the patient to follow at home to regain previous levels of fitness.
- Mental health support for symptoms of low mood, fears, frustration and problems with memory and concentration.

The rehabilitation team are able to access patient data, and thus able to monitor patients and deliver care remotely.

Other online platforms

There is a need for further online platforms for rehabilitation and recovery from long COVID syndrome. Many private health care providers have begun trialling online rehabilitation for long COVID syndrome patients — these platforms would need evaluating in the near future.

Models of telehealth rehabilitation have been studied in Australia, and a 6-week rehabilitation programme supported via telehealth was trialled in a small number of patients. In the United States, Johns Hopkins University offers telemedicine therapy, as well as appointments, to patients for rehabilitation from long COVID syndrome.

Given that long COVID syndrome is a relatively new condition, further research into these new online platforms is warranted to evaluate and compare their effectiveness in supporting the rehabilitation and recovery of patients with long COVID syndrome, so to improve their quality of life.

Key Points

- 'Your COVID Recovery' is an online rehabilitation platform widely used in the NHS in the UK; it has been expanded and updated since its launch.
- It is estimated that 10% of long COVID syndrome patients will require supervised treatment via the 'Your COVID Recovery' online platform, while 10% will benefit from digital app support for self-management.
- Many new online platforms are being trialled for rehabilitation and recovery of patients with long COVID syndrome, with further research and evaluation warranted.

References

1. NHS England and NHS Improvement (2020). Post-COVID syndrome (long COVID). Available from: https://www.england.nhs.uk/coronavirus/post-covid-syndrome-long-covid/.

2. NHS England (2021). Long COVID: the NHS plan for 2021/22. Version 1, June 2021. Available from: https://www.england.nhs.uk/coronavirus/wp-content/uploads/sites/52/2021/06/C1312-long-covid-plan-june-2021.pdf.

3. NHS England. Your COVID Recovery. Supporting your recovery after COVID-19. Available from: https://www.yourcovidrecovery.nhs.uk/.

4. Singh S. Ground breaking online COVID-19 rehab service launched. Available from: https://le.ac.uk/research/stories/human-health/covid-rehab.

5. Wootton SL, King M, Alison JA, *et al.* COVID-19 rehabilitation delivered via a telehealth pulmonary rehabilitation model: a case series. *Respirol Case Rep* 2020; 8: e00669.

6. John Hopkins Medicine. COVID-19 rehabilitation resources. Available from: https://www.hopkinsmedicine.org/physical_medicine_rehabilitation/coronavirus-rehabilitation/.

Chapter 26

Patient education and explanation

Introduction

The Scottish Intercollegiate Guidelines Network (SIGN), in collaboration with the National Institute for Health and Care Excellence (NICE) and the Royal College of General Practitioners (RCGP), published an information booklet in December 2020 (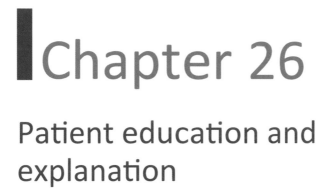 Figure 26.1), aimed at educating patients

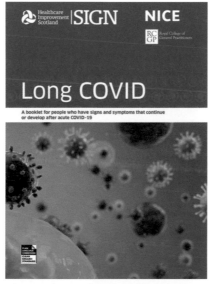

Figure 26.1. SIGN publication on long COVID for patients.

who suffer from long COVID syndrome. Patient education is a vital element aiding in recovery from illness, all the more important in the context of the COVID-19 pandemic which has caused significant global changes to all ways of life.

Fear of the unknown

Long COVID syndrome is a relatively new condition, that clinicians and health care professionals in general still poorly understand. COVID-19 illness has caused dramatic loss of human life worldwide and affected people's livelihoods. It has had a devastating impact on society and the economy. The World Health Organization (WHO) predicted that nearly half of the world's global workforce of 3.3 billion people are at risk of losing their livelihoods, while many millions are at risk of falling into extreme poverty. Fear of death and the unknown has impacted significantly on human life. Persistence of symptoms in long COVID syndrome and the sequelae of acute COVID-19 illness can cause significant catastrophisation (abnormal or exaggerated fear) and can affect the quality of life of these patients.

Patient-centred rehabilitation

Supported self-management is key to the patient-centred rehabilitation process. Thus, it is vital that patients are engaged actively in the management plan. To achieve active patient engagement in their rehabilitation, myths about long COVID syndrome should be debunked and sinister red flag symptoms ruled out, which would facilitate patient education, as well as build patient rapport.

Record keeping and patient diary

Clinicians should engage with patients in setting realistic goals, while providing guidance and support on how to achieve them. Maintaining a diary of symptoms and progress (preferably via a symptom-tracking app) will help patients with self-feedback and taking control of their management.

Explanation of the pathways

Patients with persistent symptoms of long COVID syndrome are managed via three different pathways (see Chapter 23): support in primary care, referral to multidisciplinary assessment services and referral to specialist care if there are any complications. Patients should be informed of the reasons for their referral to a particular pathway, as well as how they should engage actively in their management plan, so they clearly understand the goals and expectations from the pathway. An open, honest discussion that allows patients to participate in the process leads to their successful engagement and allows them to take control of their own recovery.

Explanation of prognosis and future

There are no research data as yet on the long-term prognosis of long COVID syndrome. While most patients recover, some may take a longer time to do so. Giving patients positive messages, as well as reassurance that sinister causes have been ruled out, is crucial in supporting patient recovery. Clinicians should explain that some symptoms might recur and disappear, but also should reassure patients that they will receive appropriate support if required, based on their needs and the severity of their condition.

Patient engagement in using rehabilitation apps

Clear and adequate information is key to engaging patients in supported self-management of long COVID syndrome. To this effect, the NHS has set up self-management apps and platforms, including the 'Your COVID Recovery' online platform.

Patient education is an important part of the recovery process, so patients can access appropriate support when needed. The 'Your COVID Recovery' online platform gives patients, as well as friends and families, detailed information on the condition to help them better understand long COVID syndrome and how to manage the condition's associated problems with a positive mindset.

Key Points

- Patient education is vital in recovery from long COVID syndrome.
- SIGN has published a patient booklet on long COVID syndrome.
- Fear of the unknown can hinder the rehabilitation process; education can help in this regard.
- 'Your COVID Recovery' is an online rehabilitation platform that facilitates patient education on rehabilitation and recovery.

References

1. Scottish Intercollegiate Guidelines Network (2020). Long COVID: a booklet for people who have signs and symptoms that continue to develop after acute COVID-19. Available from: https://www.sign.ac.uk/media/1825/sign-long-covid-patient-booklet-v2.pdf.

2. World Health Organization (2020). Impact of COVID-19 on people's livelihoods, their health and our food systems. Available from: https://www.who.int/news/item/13-10-2020-impact-of-covid-19-on-people's-livelihoods-their-health-and-our-food-systems.

3. NHS England. Your COVID Recovery — Supporting your recovery after COVID-19. Available from: https://www.yourcovidrecovery.nhs.uk.

Chapter 27

Biopsychosocial model

Introduction

Rehabilitation of patients with long COVID syndrome is based on the biopsychosocial model. COVID-19 affects individuals physically, mentally and socially. Therefore, it is prudent to adopt a holistic approach when planning for patient rehabilitation. The aim of rehabilitation should focus on improving patients' quality of life and the biopsychosocial model helps to achieve this goal.

The biopsychosocial model

Application of the biopsychosocial model (■ Figure 27.1) allows a holistic consideration of the patient based on three domains:

- 'Bio' — physiological impact of COVID-19.
- 'Psycho' — patients' altered emotions, behaviours and beliefs due to COVID-19, as well as associated catastrophisation.
- 'Social' — economic and financial, environmental, social (including family relationships), cultural and occupational impact of COVID-19.

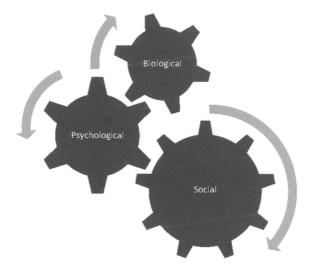

Figure 27.1. The biopsychosocial model in long COVID syndrome.

The biopsychosocial model was first proposed by George Engel in 1977 for chronic conditions and its application has been extrapolated to patients with long COVID syndrome. Health care professionals are well trained to look after the 'biological' aspect of illness, while the 'psychological' aspect can usually be explored by chronic condition specialists. However, the health care system is ill-prepared and ill-equipped in terms of tackling the 'social' impact of long COVID syndrome. It is sad that many clinicians are still unaware of the psychosocial issues arising due to long COVID syndrome, and education is needed to redress this lack of awareness.

Awareness of psychosocial issues in the COVID-19 pandemic

The COVID-19 pandemic has led to more attention on the psychosocial impact of illness on patients. An analysis study of the PubMed database showed that attention to psychological and social factors is 74% higher in COVID-19-related articles, compared to other health-related scientific articles published between January 2020 and April 2021. The author concludes that the biopsychosocial model is relevant in understanding the interrelationships among risk factors and the multidimensional clinical and psychosocial impact of COVID-19. These associations also hold true in terms of patient recovery from long COVID syndrome.

Integration of the biopsychosocial model in rehabilitation programmes

Biological, psychological and social factors all need to be considered together as a continuum. This approach will help in planning a comprehensive multidimensional, multimodal rehabilitation programme that is tailored specifically to patients' individual needs.

Importance of the biopsychosocial model in rehabilitation

It has been proposed that the biopsychosocial model can be used as the basis for new models of rehabilitation across the health and social care systems. The biopsychosocial model facilitates multidisciplinary collaboration and data sharing. It can effectively use the principle of supported self-management in patient rehabilitation where patients are encouraged to manage their recovery independently. This, in turn, would help alleviate the increasing pressures of high demands on the health care system.

Long-term benefits of the biopsychosocial model

An online narrative study of people's experiences of COVID-19 conducted over 4 months in the UK illustrated that people with a narrow range of biopsychosocial characteristics experienced a wide range of biopsychosocial impacts which are nuanced, complex and dynamic. The authors concluded that leaving these biopsychosocial issues unaddressed can lead to adverse long-term effects. In the long term, the biopsychosocial model can help reduce social and health inequalities that have been deepened as a result of the COVID-19 pandemic.

Controversies and arguments

Some groups have rejected the use of cognitive behavioural therapy and graded exercise therapy. The ME Association has been strongly against these interventions, arguing that graded exercises can be harmful in patients with long COVID syndrome (due to potential post-exertional malaise in susceptible patients).

Social media platforms have brought together thousands of patients with long COVID syndrome, thus disrupting the traditional 'authority' framework where doctors or other health care professionals are always the experts. Some patients have argued that the psychological impact of long COVID syndrome should not be stigmatised or ignored, while the organic illness should be investigated. Many claim that the voices of patients with long COVID syndrome are not being heard — constituting a form of 'structural iatrogenesis' where patients are harmed due to power imbalances that are deeply rooted in the traditional medical system.

Patients may have experienced cognitive dissonance in confronting health care structural biases. There is no way that we can progress in the management of long COVID syndrome, unless affected patients, health care professionals, managers and political leaders work together to solve the complex problem of long COVID syndrome that will affect society, as well as the economy, as a whole.

Key Points

- The biopsychosocial model is used in the rehabilitation of patients with long COVID syndrome.
- The biopsychosocial model can form the basis of new models of rehabilitation for patients with long COVID syndrome.
- The biopsychosocial model can help, in the long term, reduce social and health care inequalities that have deepened due to the COVID-19 pandemic.
- Controversies should not dampen our efforts to help patients suffering from long COVID syndrome.

References

1. Vasu T. The biopsychosocial model. In: Vasu T, Balasubramanian S, Kodivalasa M, Ingle PM. *Chronic Pain Management*, first edition. Shrewsbury: tfm Publishing Ltd; 2021, pp. 21–4.

2. Kop WJ. Biopsychosocial processes of health and disease during the COVID-19 pandemic. *Psychosom Med* 2021; 83: 304–8.

3. Engel GL. The need for a new medical model: a challenge for biomedicine. *Science* 1977; 196: 129–36.

4. Wainwright TW, Low M. Why the biopsychosocial model needs to be the underpinning philosophy in rehabilitation pathways for patients recovering from COVID-19. *Integrated Healthcare Journal* 2020; 2: e000043.

5. Stuart K, Faghy M, Bidmead E, *et al.* A biopsychosocial framework for recovery from COVID-19. *International Journal of Sociology and Social Policy* 2020; 40: 1021–39.

6. Newman M. Chronic fatigue syndrome and long COVID: moving beyond the controversy. *BMJ* 2021; 373: n1559.

7. Chew-Graham C, Lokugamage A, Simpson F (2021). How power imbalances in the narratives, research, and publications around long COVID can harm patients. Thebmjopinion. Available from: https://blogs.bmj.com/bmj/2021/06/23/how-power-imbalances-in-the-narratives-research-and-publications-around-long-covid-can-harm-patients/.

Chapter 28

Managing fatigue

Introduction

Fatigue is common after COVID-19 illness. However, in some patients, it can linger for weeks or months after the initial illness as one of the features of long COVID syndrome, causing a persistent feeling of tiredness that is exacerbated by activity and not usually relieved by rest.

It is important to strike a balance between doing gentle activity, enough to avoid the risk of deconditioning, and being overactive that could risk triggering post-activity malaise and worsening of fatigue. Finding the right balance is key to patient recovery from long COVID syndrome.

Sequelae of fatigue in long COVID syndrome

Fatigue can be a predominant symptom in long COVID syndrome. It can result in a range of sequelae that significantly affect patients' quality of life, including:

- Low levels of physical activity.
- A vicious cycle of reduced activity, worsening fatigue and muscle deconditioning.
- Poor sleep hygiene.

- Disruption of daily routine.
- Low mood, anxiety and depression.
- Feeling of unsteadiness on the feet.
- Difficulty with standing for long periods.
- Difficulty with concentration.
- Problems with memory.
- Loss of interest in life activities.

Rest and relaxation during the initial recovery period

When patients are recovering from COVID-19 illness, rest is very important, both physically and mentally. Relaxation, breathing exercises and meditation can help in this initial recovery period. Importantly, relaxation strategies should be personalised by experimenting with various methods of relaxation that would work best for the individual patient, e.g. sensory relaxation tools such as aromatherapy, including the use of essential oils, relaxing music, etc.

Being kind to self

It is important for patients to realise, and recognise, that their fatigue is real, rather than be hard on themselves. Patients, by being kind to themselves, will find it easier to understand their own fatigue, and therefore plan their activities accordingly.

Fatigue is invisible to others, and sufferers should explain their fatigue to their family, friends and colleagues so that they are aware of, and understand, the problem. Sharing the problem with others can help in resolving it. Patients should be encouraged to explain how debilitating their fatigue is, so that others understand better what the patients are going through.

Proper planning

Patients should be educated on the importance of planning their activities in advance. As in any chronic fatigue or chronic pain condition, it is important not to overdo activities and then risk being unable to do any activity later for a longer time as a consequence. In other words, avoiding a 'boom and bust cycle' can help in managing a patient's fatigue appropriately. Following a regular routine, while at the same time realising that there will be both good and bad days, can empower patients to take control of their daily living. Thus, delegating tasks and duties to family and/or colleagues, where possible, should be considered. Prioritising activities based on the patient's energy levels and time of the day can help in fatigue management.

Gradually and slowly increasing activity levels is known as 'pacing'. Pacing is key to a patient's recovery from long COVID syndrome. It involves, for example, taking an early break before the patient anticipates the need to rest. The aim is to establish a consistent pattern of activity and rest that will enable the patient to build their activity level gradually and slowly over time.

Keeping active

There is ample scientific evidence from studies on many chronic conditions that keeping active helps in patients' long-term recovery. The same principle applies to managing fatigue in long COVID syndrome. It would be sensible to use appropriate metaphors to explain to patients the importance of keeping active, but that activity levels should only be increased very slowly and gradually.

Activity diary

Patients should keep an activity diary for recording any activity, whether physical, social, emotional or cognitive. Such an activity diary will help them to understand which activities exacerbate their fatigue, and in so doing, it will help in appropriate future activity planning.

Patients should also prioritise, if possible, activities they find fun and enjoyable. It is important for patients to balance essential daily activities with fun activities, so they can become more engaged and happily participate in their recovery pathway.

Sleep hygiene

Fatigue and poor sleep hygiene are closely linked. Therefore, improving sleep hygiene can help with better fatigue management.

It is vital to keep the bedroom for sleep only, while avoiding doing anything else. Having a specific bedtime routine and ensuring the bedroom is dark can help. It is recommended to avoid spending 'screen time' (i.e. using mobile phones or other electronic devices, watching television, etc.) for at least an hour before bedtime. Avoiding caffeine intake before sleep and eating early in the evening can also help with a better sleep pattern. See Chapter 30 for more details on sleep management in long COVID syndrome.

Nutrition

Adequate nutrition and maintaining good hydration are vital in improving fatigue. This is discussed in more detail in Chapter 33.

Relaxation strategies

Deep breathing exercises can help in chronic fatigue management in long COVID syndrome. Meditation, mindfulness and complementary therapies, including acupuncture, yoga and aromatherapy, can all help with fatigue management.

Distraction strategies

Distraction strategies have been successfully used in the management of chronic conditions such as chronic pain/fatigue, including music, painting and knitting. Such strategies could also be trialled in patients suffering from long COVID syndrome.

Referral to specialist services

If fatigue does not improve after 4 weeks or worsens, or if associated with other symptoms, it would be advisable to consider referral to local long COVID, or other appropriate, specialist services.

Controversy on the use of exercise in fatigue management

The use of exercise as part of the rehabilitation programme for patients with long COVID syndrome has met with strong opposition from some patient groups, arguing that scientific evidence is equivocal on the role of exercise in managing chronic fatigue syndrome. Patients with long COVID syndrome have found it difficult to engage in standard exercise programmes, meaning they need an individually tailored, 'slow-paced' programme. Physiotherapists have acknowledged that recovery from long COVID syndrome can be slower than expected, based on their experience in treating patients with other chronic conditions.

Post-exertional malaise

It is important to realise that exercise can trigger worsening of symptoms in some patients. Therefore, any activity undertaken by the patient should be done slowly and gradually, in a manner and pace that are appropriate to that particular patient's capability.

Any rehabilitation programme should include screening patients with fatigue for post-exertional malaise during their recovery. In these patients, their threshold of activity level should be established, above which a relapse of fatigue would occur. It is important to remember that not all patients with long COVID syndrome suffer from post-exertional malaise. Long COVID syndrome affects different patients differently and hence, personalised rehabilitation planning is important to optimise patient recovery.

Key Points

- Fatigue is a common symptom in long COVID syndrome.
- It is important for patients with fatigue to rest in the initial recovery period; being kind to themselves and recognising their fatigue will help patients in their recovery.
- Pacing, planning and prioritising can help patients in recovering from long COVID syndrome.
- Establishing a good sleep pattern can help patients in managing their fatigue and activity levels.
- Long COVID syndrome affects different patients differently; therefore, personalised rehabilitation planning is important in helping patients recover from long COVID syndrome.
- Some patients suffer from post-exertional malaise; appropriate screening interventions should help to identify these patients, so that suitable rehabilitation programmes can be tailored to their specific needs for a slow and gradual recovery and to prevent relapse.

References

1. NHS England. Your COVID Recovery: fatigue. Available from: https://www.yourcovidrecovery.nhs.uk/managing-the-effects/effects-on-your-body/fatigue/.
2. Royal College of Occupational Therapists. How to manage post-viral fatigue after COVID-19. Available from: https://www.rcot.co.uk/how-manage-post-viral-fatigue-after-covid-19-0.
3. Newman M. Chronic fatigue syndrome and long covid: moving beyond the controversy. *BMJ* 2021; 373: n1559.

Chapter 29

Managing breathlessness

Introduction

Breathlessness is a common distressing symptom in patients with long COVID syndrome. Patients with long COVID syndrome can present with different degrees of breathlessness, on a background of persistent low-level infection or inflammation. Breathlessness causes significant fear and apprehension in these patients who should be given reassurance so they can engage in rehabilitation. It is also vital to rule out other sinister or treatable causes of breathlessness.

Explaining breathlessness to patients

Breathlessness is a common feature during acute COVID-19 illness, as well as in the recovery period. Supporting patients in their anxiety related to breathlessness is crucial to their engaging in rehabilitation.

Ruling out sinister or treatable causes of breathlessness

If breathlessness does not settle within a few weeks post-COVID-19 infection, it might be necessary to perform appropriate investigations such as a chest X-ray or computed tomography of the lungs. Not everyone will require further tests — the need for, and type of, investigations will depend on patient progress and/or worsening of symptoms. Pulse oximetry to monitor oxygen saturations is a non-invasive way to assess for the presence of lung damage; home pulse oximetry has been found to be a useful tool in long-term symptom management. Respiratory rate, adequacy of breathing, dyspnoea and use of accessory muscles are all useful indicators of the severity of lung damage.

It is essential to exclude cardiac causes for breathlessness, as thrombotic and cardiac complications are important differential diagnoses in post-COVID presentations.

Oxygen desaturation (i.e. below 93%, if this is new for the patient), heart rate of <60 or >100 bpm and respiratory rate of >30 breaths per minute should trigger proper assessment and investigations to rule out sinister causes through referral to appropriate acute care pathways.

Pacing and planning

Physical exertion can cause breathlessness, so it is important to pace and plan activities during recovery from long COVID syndrome. Finding the right balance between rest and activity is vital in managing breathlessness — this will vary between each patient. Therefore, patient management should be personalised by letting the patient take control of their own recovery plan, while guided by the clinician. Thus, the overall aim is self-management rehabilitation.

Breaking down individual activities into smaller chunks helps make tasks more manageable. Advance activity planning for each day of the week helps in spreading activities across the week, thus helping in energy management to control breathlessness.

Breathing control technique

Calm abdominal breathing helps towards conserving energy and requires less effort to aid breathing. The patient is asked to sit in a relaxed position on a chair, and to put one hand on the chest and the other hand on the abdomen. The patient is then asked to breathe in slowly through the nose and to breathe out through the mouth in a relaxed manner. Controlled breathing moves the hand placed on the abdomen, rising with inspiration and falling with expiration. Patients are guided to take twice as long for expiration than for inspiration, or even longer depending on their breathing pattern, symptoms and response. Combining controlled breathing with a mindfulness approach, by focusing on thoughts to release stress/tension along with breathing, will also help towards relaxation. Gentle, gradual breathing movements help in this process.

Various apps, such as Breathe2Relax, are freely available online and can be signposted to patients.

Other breathing strategies

Pursed lip breathing

This technique involves the patient breathing in through the nose and breathing out gently through the mouth, with their lips pursed, like blowing a candle or whistling. Here, expiration is longer than inspiration. This can be done during any physical activity, including walking.

Blow as you go

During an activity that requires physical exertion, e.g. going up the stairs, the patient is asked to breathe in and then to breathe out 'as they go'.

Paced breathing

Pacing breathing with activity can be helpful. For example, when climbing stairs, the patient breathes in on making one step and breathes out on making the next step.

Posture and breathlessness

Patients can adopt a position that will reduce the effort of breathing, which, in turn, would help reduce breathlessness, e.g. supporting the arms, rather than gripping them. Some patients find dropping their shoulders might help with their breathing. Leaning forward might reduce the work done by the upper body and thus also help with breathlessness.

Management of cough

It is prudent to exclude pleurisy, pneumonia or significant lung scarring as a result of acute infection, which could persist in some patients. Some long COVID patients can develop dysfunctional breathing due to deconditioning and reduced respiratory muscle strength, exacerbated by fatigue. Simple breathing control exercises can help in these situations.

Any cough that persists for >6 weeks is termed chronic cough.

Dry cough

Patients should be advised to keep well hydrated, as well as to take small sips of liquid or swallow repeatedly when starting to cough. Steam inhalation is also useful in managing dry cough, as is avoiding smoking and exposure to irritating smells.

Cough with phlegm

Patients should be advised to keep hydrated and to use steam inhalation. Breathing control exercises should also be recommended. Patients lying on their side can help with draining phlegm and reducing irritation.

Key Points

- Breathlessness is a distressing symptom in patients with long COVID syndrome; it is, however, also important to rule out other sinister or treatable causes.
- Pacing and activity planning can help to minimise breathlessness.
- Breathing control exercises and other breathing strategies are part of the management plan for breathlessness.
- Chronic cough can be managed by breathing control exercises, hydration and steam inhalation.

References

1. Your COVID Recovery. Breathlessness. Available from: https://www.yourcovidrecovery.nhs.uk/managing-the-effects/effects-on-your-body/breathlessness/.

2. Breathe2Relax app. Available from: https://play.google.com/store/apps/details?id=org.t2health.breathe2relax&hl=en_GB&gl=US.

3. Henderson R (2021). Long COVID: ongoing respiratory problems. Available from: https://www.nursinginpractice.com/clinical/respiratory/long-covid-ongoing-respiratory-problems/.

4. NHS inform. Longer-term effects of COVID-19 (long COVID). Available from: https://www.nhsinform.scot/illnesses-and-conditions/infections-and-poisoning/coronavirus-covid-19/coronavirus-covid-19-longer-term-effects-long-covid.

Chapter 30

Managing sleep

Introduction

Sleep is important for maintaining good physical and mental health. Long COVID syndrome can cause a variety of sleep disturbances, ranging from insomnia to hypersomnia. Some neurologists have termed this phenomenon of increased COVID-related sleep disturbances as 'COVID-somnia', and others 'coronasomnia'. It is clear and evident that clinicians are struggling to help those patients suffering from COVID-related sleep difficulties that significantly affect quality of life.

Sleep problems in long COVID syndrome

Hospital stay, particularly in intensive care, has a detrimental impact on sleep in the long term, mainly due to noisy environments and changes in the circadian rhythm associated with the hospital setting. Further, many medications can affect sleep, with possible long-term side effects. COVID-related effects on the central nervous system can persist in patients with long COVID syndrome.

Lack of natural daylight is known to affect the production of melatonin in the body, which is seen commonly in people with sleep problems.

Sleep disturbances can also occur during the recovery period in individuals with COVID-19 who have not been admitted to hospital. Many symptoms associated with long COVID syndrome, including breathlessness, chest discomfort, fatigue and cough, can cause sleep disruption in these patients.

Fear, anxiety and social isolation, as well as night terrors and post-traumatic stress disorder, have also exacerbated sleep problems in patients with long COVID syndrome.

Insomnia and oversleeping

Various sleep disturbances have been reported in patients with long COVID syndrome. Insomnia and disturbed sleep are commonly seen. Some patients suffer from oversleeping, as well as intense fatigue and tiredness.

When managing sleep in patients with long COVID syndrome, it is important to focus on sleep quality, and not just on sleep duration. Sleep and fatigue are closely linked, with both forming a vicious cycle that needs to be broken to aid sleep management and, in turn, recovery from long COVID syndrome.

Strategies before bedtime

Patients should be strongly advised to avoid tea, coffee, alcohol or energy drinks in the evening, and to take meals at least 2 hours before going to bed. Patients should avoid aerobic or strenuous exercises for at least 2 hours before bedtime.

There is evidence for the use of relaxation strategies, in particular breathing exercises, in improving sleep initiation. Gentle stretching and yoga have also been found to be useful to help initiate sleep. By contrast, sleeping pills often have side effects and can affect the daytime routine and worsen fatigue.

Meditation has huge positive effects in improving sleep; it uses the principles of a mindfulness-based approach, as well as lowers the neurotransmitters in the sympathetic nervous system that can cause sleep disturbances.

It is also advisable to avoid exposure to news programmes, including on social media, late in the evening, especially during the pandemic, that would risk causing significant stress, and activating the nervous system and stimulating the brain just before going to sleep.

Sleep time and sleep hygiene

Avoiding screen time before going to bed is vital, including the use of mobile phones, tablets, laptops, television and other digital devices. Maintaining regular bed times (both going to bed and waking up times) is also strongly recommended. It is important for individuals not to worry about sleeplessness in bed, as this can worsen the situation. Listening to calm music or reading a book before sleep might help. The room has to be quiet, with minimal ambient light. The bedroom temperature should not be too warm, but slightly cold.

If an individual wakes up in the middle of the night and stays awake for more than 20–30 minutes, they should be advised to get out of bed and leave the bedroom, rather than staying sleepless in bed. They can do some relaxation activities, e.g. listening to music, before returning to bed when they feel tired. It is not advisable to do, for example, work-related activities or to use a laptop in bed. The bedroom should be associated with sleeping only, as it helps set the mind for proper sleep.

Blue light filter

It has been suggested that blue light from electronic screens can suppress the production of melatonin. Most newer versions of mobile phones make use of a blue light filter to reduce eye strain and improve sleep pattern. Scientific evidence, however, is still not clear and the true effect of blue light remains debatable. In summary, it is advisable to avoid the use of mobile phones or tablets in bed and at least an hour before going to sleep.

Proper planning

It is recommended to wake up at the same time every morning, even during holiday times, to maintain a regular sleep pattern. Avoiding afternoon or daytime naps can help towards having a good night's sleep. It is not advisable to go to bed feeling hungry or thirsty.

Cognitive behavioural therapy

In severe cases of sleep deprivation, patients can be referred for psychological therapies, including cognitive behavioural therapy (CBT). In the UK, CBT for insomnia (CBT-i) is available via Improving Access to Psychological Therapies (IAPT) programmes.

Mindfulness and acceptance and commitment therapy (ACT) have been trialled in patients with long COVID syndrome to improve mental health, as well as sleep. The NHS in the UK has sleep clinics to which patients with sleep disorders can be referred for specialist treatments.

Post-traumatic stress disorder

In many patients, COVID-19 illness causes a significant physical and mental impact. Nightmares due to post-traumatic stress disorder can significantly affect sleep quality. Treatment should be based on an individualised approach for each patient. Some patients may be managed with guidance and education only, whereas others may need specialist psychological treatments.

Role of melatonin

Melatonin improves the circadian rhythm and has traditionally been used in the treatment of sleep disorders and chronic pain problems. Some researchers have trialled the use of oral melatonin to improve sleep in long

COVID patients. Evidence of its efficacy in treating sleep problems in long COVID syndrome is still awaited.

Is good sleep the answer to preventing long COVID syndrome?

It is established that recovery from long COVID syndrome is associated with improved sleep. It may not be an exaggeration to say that proper sleep could help in preventing long COVID syndrome, although it is clear that this is a 'chicken and egg' situation. Nevertheless, it would be prudent to focus on treating sleep problems as part of a multimodal approach to recovery in long COVID syndrome.

Key Points

- Sleep disturbances are common in long COVID syndrome, ranging from insomnia to hypersomnia, and result in tiredness and fatigue on waking up.
- Management should focus on sleep quality, and not only on sleep duration.
- Good sleep hygiene, avoiding the use of electronic devices in bed and associating the bedroom environment only with sleeping are vital strategies in managing sleep problems.
- Focusing on sleep management is an essential component of a multimodal approach to recovery in long COVID syndrome.

References

1. Hurley D (2020). Sleep neurologists call it 'COVID-somnia' — increased sleep disturbances linked to the pandemic. Neurology Today. Available from: https://journals.lww.com/neurotodayonline/fulltext/2020/07090/sleep_neurologists_call_it.1.aspx.

2. UC Davis Health (2020). COVID-19 is wrecking our sleep with coronasomnia — tips to fight back. Available from: https://health.ucdavis.edu/health-news/newsroom/covid-19-is-wrecking-our-sleep-with-coronasomnia--tips-to-fight-back-/2020/09.

3. Your COVID Recovery. Sleeping well. Available from: https://www.yourcovidrecovery.nhs.uk/your-wellbeing/sleeping-well/.

Chapter 31

Managing memory problems

Introduction

Brain fog is commonly described by patients suffering from long COVID syndrome. It is a vague term and is characterised by memory problems, poor concentration, feeling mentally sluggish and lack of mental clarity.

It could be a result of the effects of SARS-CoV-2 on the brain, but it also could be due to mental/mood problems, poor sleep, loneliness due to social isolation, fatigue and drug side effects.

A Norwegian study of 13,000 participants showed that 11% of SARS-CoV-2-infected patients reported memory problems (compared to 2% of untested randomly selected participants). A study from the UK of >80,000 patients post-acute COVID illness showed significant cognitive impairment of varying severity that persisted for many months in the recovery phase.

Sequelae of memory problems in long COVID syndrome

Memory problems can affect patients' ability to make decisions, as well as their concentration, which, in turn, leads to loss of confidence in doing even simple daily tasks. Patients have impaired organisational skills and become distracted, resulting in difficulty with executive functioning, which is further exacerbated by fatigue, fear and depression.

Domains of neuropsychological deficits

Studies have revealed neuropsychological deficits in attention, memory and executive functioning domains following COVID-19 illness. Cognitive deficits have been shown to be associated with anxiety and depression.

A study from the UK showed that patients with long COVID syndrome had impaired cognitive functions, including reasoning, problem-solving, spatial planning and target detection, with simpler functions spared, including working-memory span and emotional processing. These findings correlate with reports of common features of 'brain fog' such as difficulty with concentration and finding correct words.

Acceptance of memory problems

Memory problems are common during recovery from long COVID syndrome. It is important for patients to recognise and accept they have memory difficulties, so they can commit to their individualised management plans tailored specifically for their needs. Otherwise, patients will develop frustration, anger and depression. Giving reassurance and explaining that memory problems are common in long COVID syndrome can help patients to come to terms with their condition and therefore manage it appropriately.

Pacing and planning

It is possible that patients can only do one task at a time to avoid distraction. Explaining the patient's difficulty with memory to friends, family and work colleagues can help plan appropriate support to aid their recovery.

Relaxation

Calm music, yoga, meditation, breathing exercises and a mindfulness-based approach can help with relaxation, leading to better organisation and planning. Trying to make chores interesting might engage patients more with their activities.

Sleep hygiene and adequate rest

Having good sleep will improve patients' fatigue and memory problems. Appropriate planning for adequate rest in between activities can help patients considerably in managing their condition. See Chapter 30 for more details on managing sleep problems.

Nutrition

Eating a well-balanced, healthy diet helps in patient recovery from chronic conditions. See Chapter 33 for more details.

Keeping a diary and work scheduling

Keeping a diary, possibly through using a personal phone reminder function, can help in organising patients' activities. In the initial period of recovery, patients need to be kind to themselves, as well as pace themselves in their daily routine. A gradual build-up of physical and mental/emotional activities is recommended.

Association with long-term problems

Studies have suggested a possible link between long COVID syndrome and Alzheimer's disease. A small study from Argentina found such an association in the elderly population, with the risk of Alzheimer's disease being higher with persistent anosmia. However, more robust research is needed in this area before any definite conclusions are drawn.

Key Points

- Brain fog is commonly reported in long COVID syndrome.
- Recognising and accepting the problem of brain fog, proper planning and pacing can help in patient recovery from long COVID syndrome.
- Maintaining a diary and work scheduling can help in managing brain fog.

References

1. Soraas S, Bo R, Kalleberg KT, *et al.* Self-reported memory problems 8 months after COVID-19 infection. *JAMA Netw Open* 2021; 4: e2118717.

2. Almeria M, Cejudo JC, Sotoca J, *et al.* Cognitive profile following COVID-19 infection: clinical predictors leading to neuropsychological impairment. *Brain Behav Immun Health* 2020; 9: 100163.

3. Hampshire A, Trender W, Chamberlain SR, *et al.* Cognitive deficits in people who have recovered from COVID-19. *EClinicalMedicine* 2021; 39: 101044.

4. Your COVID Recovery. Memory and concentration. Available from: https://www.yourcovidrecovery. nhs.uk/managing-the-effects/effects-on-your-mind/memory-and-concentration/.

5. Erausquin GA, Gonzalez-Aleman G, *et al.* (2021). Olfactory dysfunction and chronic cognitive impairment following SARS-CoV-2 infection in a sample of older adults from the Andes mountains of Argentina. Poster presentation. 2021 Alzheimer's Association International Conference. Available from: https://alz.confex.com/alz/2021/meetingapp.cgi/Paper/57897.

Chapter 32

Managing mental health and mood problems

Introduction

As mentioned in Chapter 13, mental illness, particularly anxiety, is strongly linked to long COVID syndrome. This chapter will elaborate on management strategies for long COVID syndrome-related mental illness.

Patient self-management

The goal of rehabilitation in long COVID syndrome, including for associated mental health, is supported self-management. Patients should focus on:

- Relaxation strategies.
- Practising meditation.
- Lifestyle improvement through adopting healthy behaviours.
- Adequate nutrition.
- Proper sleep hygiene.
- Having a daily routine.
- Keeping active, while enjoying activities.
- Realistic goals broken down into small steps.
- Distraction strategies.
- Finding ways to keep connected with others.
- Sharing experiences with others.

- Getting as much natural light as possible and enjoying nature.
- Joining support groups.
- Keeping a mood diary.

Fear and anxiety

The commonest emotional responses to COVID-19 are fear and anxiety, the extent of which is significantly heightened in those with long COVID syndrome. This is mainly due to fear of the unknown when faced with symptoms persisting in the long term. Appropriate strategies that could help allay patients' fear and anxiety include:

- Breaking down problems into those that can be controlled and those that cannot; managing problems that can be controlled, rather than worrying about those that cannot be, could be helpful.
- Planning and pacing.
- Changing routines to include activities that patients are able to manage.
- Keeping note of activities that patients are able to do, to help them feel a sense of achievement.

Dealing with loss and bereavement

COVID-19 has caused significant loss of lives and many patients have experienced grief. It is even more difficult for those who are socially isolated and did not have the opportunity to grieve properly. Dealing with loss and bereavement is important in patient recovery and rehabilitation.

Pathways for mental health support

Long COVID syndrome affects various organs in different ways. Similarly, mental health problems can also present in different ways and the needs of patients with mental illness can change over time. The clinician needs to constantly review the need for mental health support and use every patient contact as an opportunity to query the patient about their mental health.

There are a range of mental health support pathways:

- Many patients self-manage with adequate education and support.
- Some patients need appropriate guidance on self-help and lifestyle modifications.
- Some patients require talking therapies and support from the local community.
- Some patients are referred to a multidisciplinary specialised group support programme.
- A small proportion of patients are referred for specialist psychological support.

Self-help strategies

Patients should be encouraged to join self-help groups and use 'recovery' apps that are dedicated to supporting patients with long COVID syndrome. Equally helpful is the 'Your COVID Recovery' platform available in the UK.

Talking about mental health

It is important to talk about mental health. COVID-19 illness is highly stressful for patients, with a significant impact on their mental health as a result of physical illness, but also due to many other factors, including social isolation, fear of the unknown, lockdown constraints, post-traumatic stress disorder and the use of personal protective equipment. It is vital that patients talk to their friends and family and/or seek emotional support from appropriately trained professionals. General practitioners should always ask their patients about their mental health when they suspect patients are experiencing long COVID syndrome.

Improving access to psychological therapies

Improving Access to Psychological Therapies (IAPT) is an initiative set up in the UK that provides talking therapies by trained specialists to which patients can be referred by their general practitioners. The use of IAPT services should be encouraged during the COVID pandemic, which would allow appropriate timely referrals to be made for patient support in the local community.

Cognitive behavioural therapy

Cognitive behavioural therapy (CBT) has been found to be effective in patients requiring coping strategies. CBT is based on changing the way patients think and behave.

Thoughts, feelings and behaviour are closely interrelated, and negative thinking can result in a vicious cycle. CBT explores these interlinks, with the aim to change these negative patterns. With CBT, problems related to long COVID syndrome are broken down into small parts, so patients develop the confidence necessary to deal with each part in a positive way. See Chapter 43 for more details on individual psychological therapies.

Acceptance and commitment therapy

While the CBT approach is based on how to control thoughts, feelings and behaviour, acceptance and commitment therapy (ACT) involves accepting and embracing the problems and committing to recovery from these difficulties. ACT is based on the relational frame theory, which proposes that rational skills may not be effective in dealing with psychological problems which should be accepted as normal and individuals need to learn healthier ways of living. ACT uses mindfulness-based approaches discussed below, and commonly involves the use of metaphors to engage patients in the acceptance pathway. See Chapter 43 for more details on individual psychological therapies.

Mindfulness-based approaches

Mindfulness involves focusing on the present moment, rather than dwelling on multiple problems and catastrophising. It is based on the use of meditation techniques and breathing strategies to achieve this goal. By focusing on the present moment, in particular on the senses of touch, sight, sound, taste and smell, this approach creates awareness of thoughts in the present moment.

Multimodal strategies in rehabilitation

It is easy to focus on recovery from physical illness and overlook mental and emotional recovery. It is important to recognise that long COVID syndrome can significantly affect mood. Therefore, proper assessment is needed so patients can be given appropriate support targeting their recovery from emotional problems as a result of long COVID syndrome.

Urgent referral for mental health support

In some cases, patients might need urgent referral for mental health. Therefore, clinicians should be aware of appropriate referral pathways for specialist mental health services. In the UK, there is a crisis helpline managed by the community mental health team in response to mental health emergencies following urgent patient referrals.

Group therapy

Group therapy has been shown to be effective in the management of many chronic conditions. It is provided as part of rehabilitation programmes for patients with long COVID syndrome, although available in only a few specialist centres. Peer support has also been shown to have significant benefit in these rehabilitation programmes.

Support to family

Long COVID syndrome affects not only the patients themselves, but also their families and/or carers, both emotionally and mentally. Burnout has been reported by family members who might find themselves feeling helpless with their loved ones suffering from long COVID syndrome. Fear of the unknown can further provoke excessive worrying. It is therefore essential to educate families and carers, so they can take active part in supporting their loved ones with problems related to long COVID syndrome, including fatigue and emotional problems.

Psychiatric referral

For patients who have significant depression or anxiety and do not seem to respond to psychological interventions, it might be appropriate to consider referral to the community mental health team for input from a psychiatrist. Some patients may also need a trial of antidepressants for their condition.

Going back to work

Social isolation and lockdown as a result of the pandemic have significantly changed the way we work. Financial pressures, including the need to rely on the furlough scheme (a government initiative in the UK for providing financial support to those who are unable to receive their wages as a result of the pandemic) and/or other social benefits, have added to the emotional stress caused by the pandemic. Job losses, and consequently loss of income, have affected entire families of many workers.

'Returnism', or going back to work, with easing of lockdown can have a significant impact on workers' mental health. It is important for employers to show understanding and be sympathetic, by finding ways to adapt the working environment to aid a smooth return to work for people affected by long COVID syndrome. Employers should actively involve their employees in planning their return to work that will help their recovery from long COVID syndrome.

Key Points

- Supported self-management is key in the management of long COVID syndrome, and patients should be guided on how to self-manage emotional problems.
- Most patients will need self-management strategies, as well as help in the community; a few patients may need referral to psychology or specialist services for management of their mental health problems.
- IAPT, CBT, ACT and mindfulness are some of the interventions that help with managing mental well-being of patients with long COVID syndrome.
- Going back to work can trigger emotional issues and employers should be sympathetic and involve their employees when making appropriate plans to aid their recovery.

References

1. Rethink Mental Illness. Long COVID and mental health. Available from: https://www.rethink.org/advice-and-information/living-with-mental-illness/wellbeing-physical-health/long-covid-and-mental-health/.
2. Mental Health Foundation. From lockdown to relaxation of covid rules: tips on looking after your mental health. Available from: https://www.mentalhealth.org.uk/coronavirus/looking-after-your-mental-health-we-come-out-lockdown.
3. Mental Health Foundation. Going back to the work environment. Available from: https://www.mentalhealth.org.uk/coronavirus/going-back-work-environment.

Chapter 33

Managing nutrition

Introduction

Patients with severe illnesses require adequate nutrition to recover in the convalescence period. This is particularly important in viral illnesses such as long COVID syndrome. Many patients with long COVID syndrome complain of loss of appetite, especially those who suffer from loss of taste and altered smell, shortness of breath, dry mouth, nausea and constipation. The majority suffer from malaise and fatigue, and need advice and support with regard to proper nutrition and hydration. Without balanced nutrition, recovery can be prolonged or hindered. Further, specific nutritional elements have been suggested to play a role in recovery, although there is no evidence to date to substantiate these claims and future research is thus warranted.

Balanced diet

A balanced diet high in protein and calories is important in the rehabilitation of patients with long COVID syndrome. Protein is needed for muscle rebuilding and improving the immune system. Carbohydrates are needed as an energy source for recovery. Fruits and vegetables provide essential minerals and vitamins. Adequate hydration is also important.

Enhanced diet for recovery

Viral illnesses cause catabolism and protein- and energy-rich foods are needed for recovery. This holds true also in recovery from long COVID syndrome where patients need protein-rich diets to build immunity and improve muscle strength, due to significant immunological insult caused by COVID illness.

Recommended protein-rich foods include meat, eggs, cheese, lentils, nuts, pulses, milk and fish.

Symptoms of nutritional deficiencies caused by COVID

Patients with nutritional deficiencies as a result of COVID illness can present with symptoms such as nausea and dry mouth. Patients with nausea should be advised to eat smaller portions of food at short intervals. Dry mouth, which is often due to shortness of breath, can make swallowing difficult, and patients with dry mouth should be advised to maintain adequate hydration and eat softer, moist foods. Sugar-free sweets or chewing gum might also help in relieving dry mouth.

A dietician's input is recommended for how to create a balanced and palatable diet to correct nutritional deficiencies. Oral nutritional supplement drinks can be taken in between meals to help patients meet their protein and energy needs.

Patients with fatigue and malaise should eat their meals slowly, in smaller portions and at frequent intervals.

For patients with loss of smell or taste, it is recommended to add a variety of herbs or spices to their food. Patients should be advised to be persistent in adding flavour to their food, should they still not respond to smell or taste, as these sensations might change over the course of their recovery.

Vitamins and minerals

Patients who have adequate nutrition might not need extra food supplements. In normal health, an individual should aim for five portions of fruits or vegetables (one portion equals 80g of fresh, frozen or tinned fruit or 150ml of fruit juice). It has been suggested that vitamins C and D can help in the recovery from illness, although research is still awaited. Many antioxidants have also been suggested to improve recovery outcomes in patients who have suffered viral illness.

Trials in nutrition

There are various trials on nutritional support and their role in long COVID syndrome. With a weak evidence base to date, it is too early to conclude on the superiority of any one type of diet. Therefore, the general principles of nutrition as described above remain the best strategy for patients in recovery from long COVID syndrome.

A Mediterranean-type diet has been proposed by some researchers, due to its high antioxidant content. The role of phytochemicals (thought to reduce inflammation) in nutritional support in patients recovering from long COVID syndrome is currently being investigated by researchers in the UK, as is the role of probiotics. Vegetables such as broccoli and cauliflower are rich in the antioxidant glutathione that could also have a possible role. As cytokine, as well as mast cell, release has been proposed to occur in acute COVID-19 illness, some have suggested a low-histamine diet to reduce inflammation in long COVID syndrome. Zinc and selenium have also been suggested for their anti-inflammatory role.

It might take a while, months or even years, before evidence from randomised controlled trials becomes available showing the efficacy of specific types of diet in patients recovering from long COVID syndrome. Until then, high-calorie, high-protein nutrition is encouraged, with individualised changes depending on patient symptoms and recovery response.

Key Points

- High-calorie, high-protein diets are vital in the recovery of patients from long COVID syndrome.
- Nutritional goals set for each patient with long COVID syndrome, and therefore the type of nutritional support, varies depending on patient symptoms and recovery response.
- Oral nutritional supplement drinks might be needed in between meals if adequate nutritional targets are not achieved.

References

1. Your COVID Recovery. Eating well. Available from: https://www.yourcovidrecovery.nhs.uk/your-wellbeing/eating-well/.
2. CancerNETUK. The UK phytochemical rich food and probiotic, covid virus intervention — the Phyto-v study. Available from: http://www.cancernet.co.uk/phyto-v.htm.

Chapter 34

Managing other symptoms

Introduction

Long COVID syndrome can present with a wide range of over 200 symptoms (see Chapter 15). Management should be individualised according to patients' presenting symptoms and the severity of their condition. For all patients with long COVID syndrome, supported self-management should be the long-term management goal.

Chronic, persistent pain in long COVID syndrome is discussed in Chapters 35 to 47.

Managing orthostatic hypotension

Orthostatic hypotension can be debilitating in long COVID syndrome. Given that gradual exercises and self-management are the goal of many rehabilitation programmes for patients with this condition, orthostatic hypotension can hinder patients in actively engaging in their rehabilitation.

Once investigations have been carried out and sinister causes ruled out, education and reassurance will help in engaging these patients in the rehabilitation pathway. Patients become reassured when they understand the physiology underlying their symptoms, especially during the tilt table test.

Given the important role of exercise in patient recovery, non-upright exercises, such as cycling on a recumbent bike or swimming, can be offered to patients. Adequate hydration is key, with a recommended daily intake of 2–3 litres of water for adults, along with the avoidance of caffeine and alcohol. In severe orthostatic hypotension, compression garments can be beneficial.

It is prudent to take a drug history to assess whether orthostatic hypotension could be caused by medications such as amitriptyline or opioids. In patients with postural orthostatic tachycardia syndrome (POTS) who are resistant to symptomatic and fluid treatment, volume-expanding pharmacological agents such as fludrocortisone can be trialled and treatment effects assessed.

Sympathomimetic alpha-1 agonists such as midodrine are also treatment options as they cause vasoconstriction, with increased venous return to the heart. Another pharmacological alternative is propranolol to treat palpitations and tachycardia in some patients; however, caution should be exercised as propranolol can cause hypotension.

Managing loss of smell and taste

The ability to experience food flavour requires both smell and taste sensations, both of which are affected in long COVID syndrome. Thus, food can taste bland or metallic, or even be tasteless. Long COVID syndrome can also affect a sufferer's appetite.

It is important for patients with long COVID syndrome to keep tasting food, as taste preferences can change throughout the disease course. Choosing food that patients like can help to ensure that they have their required calorie and nutrient intake.

Many patients will not need any treatment, with symptoms improving spontaneously. However, treatment should be considered in those whose impaired taste and smell sensations last beyond 2 weeks.

Mouth rinsing and gargling with water can help patients whose loss of taste is due to mouth dryness. Chewing sugar-free gums can also alleviate mouth dryness by stimulating salivation. In terms of food preferences, some people might prefer bland food if they feel nauseated, whereas others with loss of taste sensation might like to try spicy or strong-flavoured food. Patients can try hot and cold food to determine which they find preferable. Those who find their food now tastes very sweet as a result of long COVID syndrome can add citrus flavours (e.g. lemon or orange) to their food to help counteract the sweet taste sensation.

If taste and smell abnormalities are resistant to simple self-help measures, patients can be referred by their general practitioner to a speech and language therapist (SALT) for specialist advice.

Olfactory training for loss of smell

Patients who have loss of smell due to long COVID syndrome can undergo olfactory training, which consists of the patient actively sniffing four scents every day, spending around 20 seconds on each scent. For example, one technique involves deliberately sniffing the smell of roses, lemons, cloves and eucalyptus, for 20 seconds each, twice a day for at least 3 months. Olfactory training is the only intervention that has demonstrated efficacy in the recovery of smell sensation in patients with long COVID syndrome. It is thought to work through repeated stimulation of olfactory neurons which have neuroplastic properties.

Some clinics have used steroid sprays or supplements such as zinc and vitamins. Vitamin A has been suggested to improve olfactory neurogenesis. Systemic omega-3 fatty acids have also been proposed as treatment options by some researchers due to their neuro-regenerative or anti-inflammatory benefits.

A European Working Group consensus from different countries has issued guidance on the management of post-infectious olfactory dysfunction (PIOD) secondary to long COVID syndrome. The guidance does not recommend the use of antibiotics. The use of vitamin A drops is favoured by some in the Working Group, and the therapeutic role of oral steroids is under discussion. In summary, further research is needed before strong evidence-based recommendations can be generated.

Safety advice

It is essential to advise patients with abnormal taste and smell sensations as a result of long COVID syndrome that they should maintain smoke and carbon monoxide detectors in their home. They should also be advised to check food expiration dates and their nutritional intake.

Managing headache

Headaches are commonly reported in many viral illnesses, including COVID-19, both during acute infection and in recovery. Ruling out sinister causes can help to reassure patients. Headaches can also be associated with anxiety or mood disorders, light sensitivity and gastrointestinal problems, and are common in people with a history of migraine.

Stress is commonly associated with headaches, and patients suffering from stress should be counselled on relaxation strategies and deep breathing exercises (see Chapters 29 and 32). It is important for headache sufferers to avoid triggering factors such as smoking, caffeine and alcohol. Ideally, they should limit their use of, and regular dependence on, painkillers. Simple analgesia, including paracetamol and ibuprofen, can be helpful for headaches initially, but only in the short term; regular intake of these drugs can be a risk factor for triggering headaches. Acupuncture and other complementary therapies can have potential roles in treating headaches that need to be explored. Pain clinics can offer various treatment options (these will be discussed in later chapters).

Managing nausea and vomiting

Patients with long COVID syndrome can suffer from significant nausea. Sinister causes of nausea should be ruled out to reassure patients, so they can engage fully in the recovery pathway. Relaxation strategies and breathing exercises have a role in managing these patients with the advantage of no risk of side effects. Nausea and vomiting in long COVID syndrome can be related to loss of appetite and abnormal taste and smell sensations, which means these problems need to be addressed when managing nausea and vomiting (see earlier section on managing loss of smell and taste). Eating small portions at frequent intervals, rather than large meals, and adequate hydration can help in nausea management.

Antiemetics, including 5-HT3 receptor antagonists such as ondansetron, can be used for patients whose symptoms of nausea and vomiting do not settle.

Managing persistent fever

Low-grade intermittent fever has been observed in some patients with long COVID syndrome. This can cause significant fear and apprehension in affected patients. It has been suggested that persistent lymphocytosis could be associated with increases in temperature in long COVID syndrome.

It is important to rule out infections and other sinister causes. Antipyretic treatment and reassurance can help in the management of these patients.

Managing loss of appetite

One in three patients with COVID-19 suffer a loss of appetite, which can be persistent in some patients and is exacerbated by nausea, fatigue, fever and medications. Appetite loss that persists for more than a week in the recovery phase is potentially serious and should be investigated and managed appropriately.

It is important to advise patients with a loss of appetite to maintain their fluid intake and to eat small meals, rather than stop eating altogether. Patients should try different foods, as taste and smell abnormalities can change during the recovery phase. High-protein and high-energy diets are also essential.

Patients should be educated on the importance of allowing for longer mealtimes, as fatigue can be a constraint for these patients. Oral nutritional supplement drinks could be recommended in cases of insufficient calorie and protein intake. Patients with persistent appetite loss despite the measures described above should be referred to a dietician.

Managing gastrointestinal reflux

Gastrointestinal reflux has been reported in long COVID syndrome and is associated with coughing in a few patients. Once other causes of gastrointestinal reflux have been ruled out, anti-reflux medications can be used in persistent cough.

Managing tinnitus

Audiovestibular problems have been associated with COVID-19, including hearing loss (7.6%), tinnitus (14.8%) and vertigo (7.2%). Stress is also known to be associated with tinnitus and needs to be managed. With no cure available, management of tinnitus in long COVID syndrome relies on symptomatic treatment.

Managing diarrhoea

Bowel problems are commonly reported in long COVID syndrome. Loss of appetite, nausea, anxiety and stress could all be associated with bowel problems. It is prudent to first rule out treatable causes, so clinicians can then reassure patients and manage their bowel symptoms.

Managing itch and skin problems

An international registry of COVID-19 dermatological manifestations reported from 41 countries found the presence of morbilliform rash, urticarial eruptions, papulosquamous eruptions and pernio in patients with long COVID syndrome, even many days post-acute infection. For example, pernio lesions were found to persist for more than 60 days in long COVID patients.

Skin rashes require the use of moisturisers, as well as topical steroid creams if persistent. For dry skin, patients should be advised to use moisturisers, rather than soap, for showering.

In COVID digits, or COVID toes, the toes become tender and swollen, accompanied by purple discoloration. This condition can persist even 3 months post-acute illness. The use of simple analgesia can be used for pain relief.

Ulcers in the oral cavity can benefit from antiseptic lozenges and mouthwashes.

Key Points

- Orthostatic hypotension can be debilitating to patients with long COVID syndrome; appropriate education and patient-specific treatment plans are important in patient management.
- Olfactory training has been found to be helpful in patients with long COVID syndrome who suffer from abnormal smell sensation.
- More than 200 symptoms have been reported by patients with long COVID syndrome.
- Skin manifestations can persist for long periods after COVID-19 illness.

References

1. Dani M, Dirksen A, Taraborreli P, et al. Autonomic dysfunction in 'long COVID': rationale, physiology and management strategies. Clin Med 2021; 21: e63–7.
2. NHS England. Your COVID Recovery. Taste and smell. Available from: https://www.yourcovidrecovery. nhs.uk/managing-the-effects/effects-on-your-body/taste-and-smell/.

3.   Whitcroft KL, Hummel T. Olfactory dysfunction in COVID-19. Diagnosis and management. *JAMA* 2020; 323: 2512–4.

4.   Levy JM. Treatment recommendations for persistent smell and taste dysfunction following COVID-19 — the coming deluge. *JAMA Otolaryngol Head Neck Surg* 2020; 146: 733.

5.   Addison AB, Wong B, Ahmed T, *et al.* Clinical Olfactory Working Group consensus statement on the treatment of postinfectious olfactory dysfunction. *J Allergy Clin Immunol* 2021; 147: 1704–19.

6.   Arita Y, Yamamoto S, Nagata M, *et al.* Long COVID presenting with intermittent fever after COVID-19 pneumonia. *Radiol Case Rep* 2021; 16: 2478–81.

7.   ZOE COVID Study. Is a loss of appetite a symptom of COVID-19? Available from: https://covid.joinzoe.com/post/covid-symptoms-skipped-meals.

8.   Almufarrij I, Munro KJ. One year on: an updated systematic review of SARS-CoV-2, COVID-19 and audio-vestibular symptoms. *Int J Audiol* 2021; 60: 935–45.

9.   McMahon DE, Gallman AE, Hruza GJ, *et al.* Long COVID in the skin: a registry analysis of COVID-19 dermatological duration. *Lancet Infect Dis* 2021; 21: 313–4.

10.   NHS England. Your COVID Recovery. Skin disorders. Available from: https://www.yourcovidrecovery.nhs.uk/managing-the-effects/effects-on-your-body/skin-disorders/.

Section V

Pain management in long COVID syndrome

Chapter 35

Managing pain in long COVID syndrome

Introduction

Pain and fatigue are commonly reported in long COVID syndrome and can be challenging for primary care clinicians to manage. Multiple joint pain, widespread pain, muscle pain, chest pain or tightness, pins and needles, headache, earache and sore throat are some examples of chronic pain in patients with long COVID syndrome.

Joint and muscle pain

Musculoskeletal pain usually resolves in the majority of patients with long COVID syndrome but can be persistent in a minority and become debilitating. Hospital stays, restricted mobility due to comorbidities, side effects of medications, restrictions imposed by social isolation can all cause muscle deconditioning and thus exacerbate pain. In addition to pain itself, patients can also complain of weakness, tiredness and stiffness where even minimal physical activity can cause malaise and tiredness.

Widespread neuropathic sensations

Neuropathic sensations, including dysaesthesia (abnormal sensations), allodynia (touch sensations causing pain) and hyperalgesia (heightened sensitivity to painful stimuli), have been reported by patients with long COVID syndrome. Patients complain of numbness or pins and needles in a non-dermatomal or widespread pattern.

Biopsychosocial model

Nociception is only a small component of the pain experience. Pain can affect long COVID patients in various aspects of life, including their psychological ability to cope and their social life. Evidence shows that chronic pain affects the sufferer's quality of life. It is recommended to use the biopsychosocial model, so care is focused on outcome measures of the patient's quality of life, rather than on pain management alone. Most pain services apply this model in their approach to treating patients suffering with pain. For more details on the biopsychosocial model, see Chapter 27.

Multimodal strategies

Chronic pain is resistant to interventions. Treatment requires a multimodal approach, including self-management, physiotherapy, complementary therapies, simple medications, coping strategies and rehabilitation programmes. Clinicians should always set a comprehensive multimodal recovery plan when treating patients with long COVID syndrome.

Further, the combined use of multiple interventions can have a synergistic effect and thus decrease the risk of side effects from medications.

Gradual pacing

The aim of the multimodal approach is to keep active. However, a patient's level of activity can vary, depending on the severity of their long COVID symptoms and the degree of post-exertional malaise from which the patient suffers. For more details on gradual pacing, see Chapters 28 and 36.

Physical therapy

Exercise is key to patient recovery. However, importantly, the 'boom and bust cycle' should be avoided. The physiotherapist or occupational therapist will help the patient find the right balance between activity and rest, to minimise the risk of post-exertional malaise. Physiotherapists have found this to be more challenging when treating patients with long COVID syndrome, compared with treating those with other widespread pain conditions such as fibromyalgia. Patient reassurance to make them feel self-confident is important in their recovery process. It is advisable to start with low-intensity activities and those that the patient enjoys in their daily life. For more details on physical therapy, see Chapter 36.

Stretching exercises

Stretching exercises strain the muscles more than normal activities and should be cautiously done in the initial phase of rehabilitation. As patients gain confidence, these stretching exercises can be gradually increased. A slow and gradual increase is the key to patient recovery. It may be wise to start with one or two stretching sessions in the first few weeks of rehabilitation and see how the patient responds before increasing these exercises. Examples of stretching exercises include walking uphill, climbing stairs, lifting weights and working with resistance bands, all of which can be done only in the confirmed absence of post-exertional malaise or worsening of symptoms with activities.

Getting help

If symptoms worsen or if patients cannot take part in any exercise activity due to fatigue or breathlessness, it is important that they contact the primary care clinician. Patients should also seek medical help if they have new symptoms of pins and needles or worsening weakness.

Referral to specialist services

For patients who suffer from pain as well as various other systemic symptoms and are resistant to treatment, it is sensible to consider referral to local long COVID specialist services. If pain alone is the problem, and the other symptoms can be managed in primary care, patients might benefit from the help of a chronic pain consultant in the pain clinic.

Problems specific to COVID times

Most pain services have been affected due to their staff being redeployed to look after sick patients at the height of the COVID pandemic. This has led to delays in both access and referrals of long COVID patients to chronic pain services. This has, in turn, resulted in overburdened specialist pain services, which now need coordination with local rehabilitation services.

Problems due to delayed access to pain services

Delayed referrals of long COVID patients to pain clinics or specialist rehabilitation services can result in worsening of pain, disability and depression. It is essential to prioritise available resources for patients who are in the most urgent need of help. Thus, patients with the most severe restrictions due to pain and those in the most vulnerable groups should be immediately referred to pain and rehabilitation services.

Key Points

- Joint and muscle pain, widespread pain and neuropathic sensations are debilitating symptoms experienced by patients with long COVID syndrome during their recovery.
- The biopsychosocial model is a recommended approach in patient rehabilitation, and the use of multimodal strategies is advised.
- If pain is resistant to treatment in primary care, appropriate referral to specialist rehabilitation services or chronic pain services should be considered.
- Restrictions due to lockdown during the COVID pandemic and redeployment of health care resources have led to significant problems in access to specialist services.

References

1. Vasu T. The biopsychosocial model. In: Vasu T, Balasubramanian S, Kodivalasa M, Ingle PM. *Chronic Pain Management,* first edition. Shrewsbury: tfm Publishing Ltd; 2021, pp. 21–4.

2. Your COVID Recovery. Musculoskeletal, shoulder and back pain. Available from: https://www.yourcovidrecovery.nhs.uk/managing-the-effects/effects-on-your-body/musculoskeletal-shoulder-and-back-pain/.

3. Kemp HI, Corner E, Colvin LA. Chronic pain after COVID-19: implications for rehabilitation. *Br J Anaesth* 2020; 125; 436–49.

4. El-Tallawt SN, Nalamasu R, Pergolizzi JV, *et al.* Pain management during the COVID-19 pandemic. *Pain Ther* 2020; 9: 453–66.

Chapter 36

Physical therapy

Introduction

Physiotherapy is an important intervention in any rehabilitation programme. Rehabilitation enables and supports patients in their recovery or adjustment from illness, so they can achieve their full potential and live as fully and actively as possible. It is wise to start physiotherapy early, but gradually, in patients with long COVID syndrome, to avoid flare-ups of fatigue and weakness.

Role of the physiotherapist

The physiotherapist has the following roles in a patient's recovery pathway:

- To assess the extent and nature of the patient's problems.
- To determine how these problems affect their daily life, as well as quality of life.
- To examine the patient to rule out sinister or treatable causes, along with guidance from their doctor if needed.
- To set achievable realistic goals based on the patient's values.
- To educate the patient on their condition.
- To prescribe tailored exercise and activity plans for the individual patient.

- To advise on breathing exercises and demonstrate these exercises to the patient.
- To teach the patient relaxation and pacing strategies.
- To provide manual therapy treatment and support.
- To review patient progress and make further plans.
- To work as a team together with other health care professionals involved in the patient's rehabilitation.
- Some physiotherapists might add complementary therapies to the rehabilitation plan.
- Some physiotherapists also use counselling or psychological approaches.

The physiotherapist helps the patient with long COVID syndrome to gradually improve their strength and mobility, while monitoring the patient to avoid post-exertional malaise (PEM). This therapy process is more challenging in long COVID patients, compared with physiotherapy in those with other chronic conditions, as patients can easily and unpredictably suffer fatigue relapse upon simple exertion. Further, long COVID patients suffer from a range of symptoms, which are challenging for the physiotherapist to manage.

Safety first

Long COVID syndrome presents to the physiotherapist with many challenges. The main goal of the physiotherapist that is specific to this condition is to avoid post-exertional malaise (PEM) or post-exertional symptom exacerbation (PESE). If a patient complains of fatigue, it is advisable not to push them further, as this can lead to a vicious cycle resulting in more fatigue.

Therefore, it is essential for the physiotherapist to establish a good rapport with the patient and to assess them thoroughly. A good multidisciplinary team approach to assessment and communication will help in the rehabilitation of the patient.

Excluding cardiac and respiratory impairment

Cardiac problems should be excluded before starting any exercise interventions. Continued monitoring for potential delayed cardiac complications is also important during gradual exercise programmes. Patients can present with oxygen desaturation on exertion during rehabilitation. Therefore, oxygen saturation monitoring is important in symptomatic patients. The physiotherapist should remember that these patients can present with autonomic dysfunction and orthostatic hypotension, and these should be screened for before starting exercise activities.

Personalised approach

Each long COVID patient presents in a different way, as long COVID syndrome is known to be associated with more than 200 different types of symptoms. The severity and nature of long COVID symptoms vary among patients and even within each patient at different stages of their recovery. Constant assessment and review are needed. The main goal should be supported self-management.

Activity diary

Patients should maintain an activity diary, recording all activities, including physical, cognitive and emotional, and relating these to their fatigue level. By looking retrospectively at their recorded activities and their associated fatigue levels, patients will be able to plan, prioritise and pace their future activities. Physiotherapists can guide patients appropriately based on the information recorded by patients in their activity diaries.

Gradual pacing

The aim of physical therapy is to keep active. However, a patient's activity level can vary, depending on the severity of their symptoms of long COVID syndrome and the degree of PEM from which the patient suffers. For more details on pacing, see Chapter 28.

Breathing exercises and support

Chapter 29 elaborates on the techniques of breathing exercises and support. Physiotherapists have a major role in educating patients and demonstrating these exercises, as well as explaining their scientific rationale, so that patients are motivated to do them regularly. Patients with breathlessness should be advised to spend at least 10 minutes twice a day to retrain their breathing pattern in the rehabilitation process.

Using the same respiratory physiotherapy strategies as in other conditions might not be suitable in long COVID syndrome, as they can result in more fatigue and tiredness, thus significantly exacerbating patients' symptoms.

Stretching exercises

Stretching exercises strain the muscles more than normal activities and should be cautiously done in the initial phase of rehabilitation. As patients gain confidence, these stretching exercises can be gradually increased. A slow and gradual increase is the key to patient recovery. It may be wise to start with one or two stretching sessions in the first few weeks of rehabilitation and see how the patient responds before increasing these exercises. Examples of stretching exercises include walking uphill, climbing stairs, lifting weights and working with resistance bands.

Holistic approach

Physiotherapists are specialised in treating patients holistically, with patients kept at the centre of all management plans. Each plan should be individualised according to the specific symptoms from which patients suffer.

How to manage post-exertional malaise

PEM can exacerbate fatigue and tiredness, and can lead to a difficult vicious circle. Patients should be reassured and assessed to determine the precipitating factor for their PEM, their level and intensity of activity and their activity level that would be tolerable in the future.

PEM can exacerbate many other systemic symptoms in patients with long COVID syndrome. Sometimes, it is disproportionate to the triggering activity and might not be relieved by rest. Unfortunately, post-exertional worsening of symptoms is unpredictable and even many experienced physiotherapists struggle with finding the right balance in the level of activities appropriate specifically for patients with long COVID syndrome.

Rest is important in recovery from PEM. Once the trigger, as well as their triggering threshold, has been identified, patients should be reassured and advised to rest. When resuming exercises, a cautious approach should be taken, starting at a lower level than the triggering threshold identified and proceeding at a slower pace than previously. Working within patients' energy limits can be challenging and patients should be given the power to take control of their level of activities and what they are able to achieve, along with the support and encouragement from the physiotherapist.

A 'stop-rest-pace' approach is recommended in managing patients with PEM.

Safe rehabilitation approach

Various physiotherapy and patient groups published a guideline in June 2021 on the safe rehabilitation of patients with long COVID syndrome. This guideline emphasises the need for proper assessment to exclude red flags, including PEM and respiratory or cardiac problems, before planning for exercise interventions.

Key Points

- Physiotherapy is an important intervention in the rehabilitation of patients with long COVID syndrome.
- Red flag symptoms should be excluded before starting exercise programmes; cardiac or respiratory problems causing desaturation or heart rate and blood pressure changes might limit patients' exercise capacity.
- Physiotherapists should always assess patients for risks of PEM which can hinder the recovery pathway; if PEM occurs, 'stop — rest — pace' is the recommended approach.
- An individualised personal approach should be taken for each patient, as symptoms, severity and risk of post-exertional fatigue vary among patients.

References

1. Chartered Society of Physiotherapy. Rehabilitation. Available from: https://www.csp.org.uk/conditions/rehabilitation.
2. Chartered Society of Physiotherapy. What is long Covid? Available from: https://www.csp.org.uk/news/coronavirus/clinical-guidance/long-covid.
3. World Physiotherapy (2021). World Physiotherapy response to COVID-19. Briefing paper 9. Safe rehabilitation approaches for people living with long COVID: physical activity and exercise. Available from: https://world.physio/sites/default/files/2021-07/Briefing-Paper-9-Long-Covid-FINAL-English-2021_0.pdf.

Chapter 37

Massage and hot and cold therapies

Introduction

Massage therapy, heat and cold topical applications, aromatherapy and hydrotherapy have been trialled in various rehabilitation programmes. However, it is too early to recommend their use in the management of long COVID syndrome due to a lack of trials that are yet to be conducted.

Massage therapy

Massage therapy can have both physical and psychological benefits in the rehabilitation process. It offers the opportunity to educate patients on supported self-management principles as part of their rehabilitation pathway, whereby patients should be encouraged to take control of their own recovery with the use of 'passive' treatment. Scientific evidence has been lacking in the use of massage therapy in chronic conditions, such as chronic pain and arthritis, and proper evaluation of its efficacy is needed.

Massage therapy involves physical manipulation of soft tissues in the body. The Swedish or classical massage technique is usually applied in Western countries. Therapists from the Indian subcontinent use a traditional Ayurvedic massage with herbal oils that is particularly popular in Kerala and regions in South India. Other techniques include sports massage, deep tissue massage, clinical massage and Eastern techniques such as shiatsu, Thai and tuina.

Some studies have shown positive results on the use of massage therapy in generalised pain conditions such as fibromyalgia. This could be extrapolated to trialling the technique in patients with long COVID syndrome, while awaiting relevant research data.

Heat therapy

Heat therapy, or thermotherapy, involves the application of heat in various forms, such as a hot-water bottle, heat pad, ultrasound, wheat bag and electric heating pad, to help relieve pain and fatigue. It is commonly used by many patients, although scientific evidence on its efficacy is limited. Heat increases blood supply, while reducing inflammation and oedema, and can reduce stiffness and muscle spasms. Theoretically, improved blood circulation, and thereby oxygen delivery, can improve and speed up the healing process.

Heat-based therapies can offer psychological benefits by improving mental well-being, enhancing relaxation and improving sleep. The use of heat therapy is cheap, convenient and widely accessible.

Awareness of skin hygiene is essential in heat therapy to prevent skin damage. However, heat therapy is generally a harmless technique, so its application can be trialled on patients with long COVID syndrome. Many rehabilitation programmes and pain/physiotherapy services use this approach as a part of the multimodal recovery pathway.

Cold therapy

Cold therapy can be suitable for some patients. Cold temperatures slow blood flow and can reduce swelling and pain. Cold therapy can be applied, e.g. using a specially designed cold pack, a bag of frozen vegetables or ice wrapped in a towel, or even a towel soaked in cold water, over painful areas. A cold bag can be kept in the freezer to be used topically when needed.

Aromatherapy

No research is available on the use of aromatherapy in long COVID syndrome. Given that olfactory therapy is used successfully in treating loss of smell and taste in this condition (see Chapter 34 for details), trials to study the benefits of aromatherapy are warranted.

Hydrotherapy

Although hydrotherapy is used successfully in many rehabilitation programmes, it is too early to give evidence-based advice on its use in long COVID syndrome. Hydrotherapy utilises the benefits of physical properties of water such as buoyancy, hydrostatic pressure and viscosity, thereby engaging patients in a slow recovery pathway. Hydrotherapy also helps to improve mental well-being, which, in turn, further stimulates patient participation in their treatment. However, since patients with long COVID syndrome can have red flag symptoms, including cardiorespiratory symptoms or postural orthostatic intolerance, proper assessment is needed to determine the suitability of hydrotherapy in these patients.

Key Points

- Massage and hot and cold topical therapies are commonly used in many rehabilitation programmes and should be considered in the management of patients with long COVID syndrome.
- With a current lack of evidence, it is too early to give recommendations on the use of these therapeutic adjuncts.
- Supported self-management should be the goal of patient recovery, even if 'passive' therapies are used in the multimodal rehabilitation pathway.

References

1.	National Center for Complementary and Integrative Health (2019). Massage therapy: what you need to know. Available from: https://www.nccih.nih.gov/health/massage-therapy-what-you-need-to-know.
2.	Cohen M. Turning up the heat on COVID-19: heat as a therapeutic intervention. *F1000Res* 2020; 9: 292.

Chapter 38

Simple medications

Introduction

Painkillers are commonly used as part of the multimodal rehabilitation pathway in long COVID syndrome. This chapter deals with simple painkillers, including paracetamol and non-steroidal anti-inflammatory drugs (NSAIDs).

The Commission on Human Medicines (a committee of the Medicines and Healthcare products Regulatory Agency) and the National Institute for Health and Care Excellence (NICE), as well as dental guidelines, such as from the Scottish Dental Clinical Effectiveness Programme and NHS England, support the use of paracetamol and NSAIDs in COVID patients. However, there is only limited research on the use of these analgesics in patients with long COVID syndrome who are undergoing rehabilitation.

Paracetamol

Paracetamol is a simple analgesic and antipyretic drug that is available over the counter. Also known as N-acetyl-para-aminophenol, it is derived from phenol and has a core benzene ring structure. The maximum oral dose for adults is 1g taken every 4–6 hours (hence a maximum dose of 4g in 24 hours). When taken orally, the onset of its analgesic effects is within 40 minutes, peaking after 1 hour. It has a good safety profile and effectiveness.

Paracetamol inhibits prostaglandin E synthesis in the cyclo-oxygenase (COX) pathway and can also affect the nociceptive pathway. Several central and peripheral mechanisms of action have been suggested. It has an oral bioavailability of 70–90%, whereas rectal bioavailability is variable at around 40%. Paracetamol is metabolised in the liver primarily by glucuronidation. A small fraction is oxidised by cytochrome P450 enzymes to form N-acetyl-p-benzoquinone imine (NAPQI), which is a toxic metabolite in paracetamol overdose, causing liver damage due to glutathione deficiency.

There is no research on the use of paracetamol in long COVID syndrome. However, it is commonly used for musculoskeletal pain relief, especially during physiotherapy in rehabilitation.

Paracetamol can also be useful as an antipyretic in patients with long COVID syndrome who have persistent intermittent fever.

Non-steroidal anti-inflammatory drugs

NSAIDs are used in a variety of painful conditions and have also been trialled in patients with long COVID syndrome for musculoskeletal pain. They are classified as follows:

- Non-selective NSAIDs, including:
  - salicylates (aspirin);
  - acetic acid derivatives (diclofenac, ketorolac, indomethacin);
  - fenamates (mefenamic acid);
  - oxicam derivatives (meloxicam, piroxicam);
  - propionic acid derivatives (ibuprofen, naproxen).
- Selective COX-2 inhibitors, including pyrazoles (celecoxib, parecoxib, etoricoxib); these have fewer gastrointestinal side effects. Some COX-2 inhibitors (rofecoxib and valdecoxib) have been withdrawn due to their cardiovascular side effects.

Topical NSAIDs are commonly used and available over the counter (e.g. ibuprofen gel, diclofenac gel).

NSAIDs act as COX inhibitors, thereby reducing prostaglandin production; prostaglandins cause fever, pain and inflammatory responses (■ Figure 38.1).

COX-1 is constitutively expressed, mediating prostaglandin production, and is involved in gastric mucosal protection, maintenance of renal blood flow and thromboxane synthesis (involved in platelet aggregation and vasoconstriction). The main side effects of NSAIDs include gastric ulceration, renal damage and bleeding due to their inhibitory effects on COX.

COX-2 is an inducible form of the enzyme that is responsible for the production of prostaglandin E2 (PGE2), which causes inflammatory responses and pain. However, COX-2-selective NSAIDs have fewer side effects.

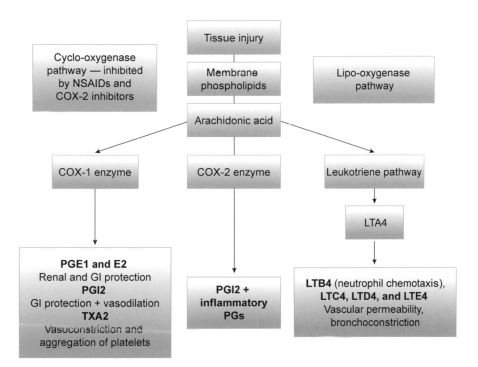

Figure 38.1. Mechanism of action of NSAIDs. COX-1 = cyclo-oxygenase-1; COX-2 = cyclo-oxygenase-2; NSAID = non-steroidal anti-inflammatory drug; PG = prostaglandin; PGE1 = prostaglandin E1; PGE2 = prostaglandin E2; PGI2 = prostaglandin I2; TXA2 = thromboxane A2; LT = leukotriene.

In addition to the above-mentioned side effects, NSAIDs can also precipitate bronchoconstriction in patients with asthma by stimulating the leukotriene pathway.

Ibuprofen should be taken at a maximum dose of 200–400mg orally 3–4 times daily on a full stomach, along with gastric protection, given its risk profile.

Key Points

- Simple painkillers, including paracetamol and NSAIDs, can be used in long COVID syndrome.
- These medications can help in relieving pain, including in rehabilitation.

References

1. National Institute for Health and Care Excellence (2020). COVID-19 rapid evidence summary: acute use of non-steroidal anti-inflammatory drugs (NSAIDs) for people with or at risk of COVID-19. Evidence summary [ES23]. Available from: www.nice.org.uk/guidance/es23.

2. Crighton AJ, McCann CT, Todd EJ, et al. Safe use of paracetamol and high-dose NSAID analgesia in dentistry during the COVID-19 pandemic. Br Dent J 2020; 229: 15–8.

3. Ingle PM. Pharmacology — simple analgesics — paracetamol. In: Vasu T, Balasubramanian S, Kodivalasa M, Ingle PM. Chronic Pain Management, first edition. Shrewsbury: tfm Publishing Ltd; 2021, pp. 219–22.

4. Ingle PM. Pharmacology — non-steroidal anti-inflammatory drugs (NSAIDs). In: Vasu T, Balasubramanian S, Kodivalasa M, Ingle PM. Chronic Pain Management, first edition. Shrewsbury: tfm Publishing Ltd; 2021, pp. 223–33.

5. Scottish Dental Clinical Effectiveness Programme (SDCEP) (2020). Management of acute dental problems during COVID-19 pandemic. Available from: https://www.sdcep.org.uk/published-guidance/acute-dental-problems-covid-19/.

6. NHS England (2020). COVID-19 guidance and standard operating procedure: for the provision of urgent dental care in primary care dental settings and designated urgent dental care provider sites. Version 3. Available from: https://www.england.nhs.uk/coronavirus/wp-content/uploads/sites/52/2020/06/C0581-covid-19-urgent-dental-care-sop-update-16-june-20-.pdf.

Chapter 39

Neuropathic pain medications

Introduction

Neuropathic pain is one of the clinical presentations of long COVID syndrome. Pharmacological agents might be needed as a part of the multimodal plan for rehabilitation and recovery of patients with this condition. There is limited evidence on the use of neuropathic pain medications in long COVID syndrome. However, based on their efficacy in treating neuropathic pain in other chronic conditions, use of these drugs is currently being trialled in patients with long COVID syndrome. Further, long COVID syndrome can also present with neurological complications, including polyneuropathy, stroke, encephalitis, myelitis and Guillain-Barré syndrome, all of which might need pharmacological therapy for neuropathic pain relief.

A few case reports have described patients with acute COVID-19 illness experiencing severe neuropathic pain. Gabapentinoids were found to be beneficial in treating pain in these patients.

Tricyclic antidepressants

Tricyclic antidepressants, including amitriptyline and nortriptyline, are the first-line choice for the management of neuropathic pain, according to the National Institute for Health and Care Excellence (NICE) guidelines. Their mechanism of action is via inhibition of presynaptic reuptake of noradrenaline and serotonin. In neuropathic pain, the number needed to treat is 3.6.

Tricyclic antidepressants are metabolised in the liver and excreted via the kidneys. They are contraindicated in arrhythmias, the manic phase of bipolar disorder, heart block and immediately post-myocardial infarction.

Side effects are anticholinergic (dry mouth, constipation, blurred vision, urinary retention), antihistaminergic (drowsiness) and anti-alpha-adrenergic (low blood pressure, prolonged QT interval and atrioventricular block).

The drugs are taken orally once daily at doses of 10–75mg. Patients should be commenced on a small dose, which is then slowly increased, as needed and depending on side effects. It is advised to take tricyclic antidepressants in the early evening to avoid drowsiness on waking up in the morning. Dry mouth can be persistent and patients should be advised regarding adequate hydration.

Gabapentinoids

Gabapentinoids bind to the α2δ (alpha-2 delta) subunit of voltage-gated calcium channels, resulting in a reduction of presynaptic calcium influx, thereby reducing the release of excitatory neurotransmitters (such as glutamate, substance P and calcitonin gene-related peptide [CGRP]) from neuronal tissues. The efficacy of gabapentinoids has not yet been studied in long COVID syndrome, although it is used by clinicians for patients with long COVID syndrome and has been reported in case reports.

Pregabalin is more potent than gabapentin. Pregabalin has a better pharmacokinetic profile, as well as better bioavailability and a longer duration of action, compared to gabapentin. In neuropathic pain, the number needed to treat for gabapentinoids is 4.2–6.4.

Central nervous system side effects, pedal oedema, increased body weight and gastrointestinal side effects are common with the use of gabapentinoids.

Gabapentin is taken orally and started at 300mg once daily, then increased gradually, up to a usual dose of 600mg three times daily. Smaller doses can be trialled if there are side effects. Pregabalin is taken orally and started at 25mg or 75mg once daily, depending on the patient's weight, and increased gradually, up to a maximum dose of 300mg twice daily. After a trial of 4–6 weeks, if gabapentinoids have not helped, patients should be gradually weaned off them. Starting low and going slow is the key to success in drug therapy for chronic pain.

In the UK, due to potential misuse, these drugs are classified as class C controlled drugs, meaning they are available only on prescription issued by a qualified health care professional.

Serotonin and noradrenaline reuptake inhibitors

Serotonin and noradrenaline reuptake inhibitors (SNRIs), such as duloxetine, are used in the treatment of neuropathic pain, but are less studied in long COVID syndrome. They inhibit presynaptic serotonin and noradrenaline reuptake. In neuropathic pain conditions, the number needed to treat is 6.4. SNRIs are usually taken orally and started at a dose of 30–60mg once daily, which is then increased to a maximum dose of 120mg daily. Side effects include sleep problems, headache, dizziness, blurred vision and dry mouth.

NICE guidelines for neuropathic pain

NICE guidance on neuropathic pain before the COVID-19 pandemic recommends the use of amitriptyline, gabapentin, pregabalin or duloxetine. If initial treatment with one drug is not effective, another drug from the list should be used. For acute rescue therapy, the guidance recommends the use of tramadol, and capsaicin cream for localised neuropathic pain.

There is currently only limited evidence on the use of neuropathic pain medications in long COVID syndrome. Therefore, it is prudent to use the usual principles of neuropathic pain management in patients with long COVID syndrome, including the multimodal biopsychosocial approach. Overall, after a trial of 4–6 weeks of drug treatment, it is important to review the patient to assess the efficacy and side effects of the treatment.

Key Points

- There is currently limited evidence on the use of neuropathic pain medications in long COVID syndrome, although these are being used by clinicians since neuropathic pain is a common presentation of the condition.
- Neuropathic pain medications are used as per NICE clinical guidelines, and the use of amitriptyline and gabapentinoids has been reported in patients with long COVID syndrome.

References

1. Attal N, Martinez V, Bouhassira D. Potential for increased prevalence of neuropathic pain after the COVID-19 pandemic. *Pain Rep* 2021; 6: e884.

2. Aksan F, Nelson EA, Swedish KA. A COVID-19 patient with intense burning pain. *J Neurovirol* 2020; 10: 1–2.

3. National Institute for Health and Care Excellence (2013). Neuropathic pain in adults: pharmacological management in non-specialist settings. Clinical guideline [CG173]. Available from: https://www.nice.org.uk/guidance/cg173.

4. Murally H, Ingle PM. Pharmacology — other anti-neuropathic agents. In: Vasu T, Balasubramanian S, Kodivalasa M, Ingle PM. *Chronic Pain Management*, first edition. Shrewsbury: tfm Publishing Ltd; 2021, pp. 255–62.

5. Ingle PM. Pharmacology — gabapentinoids. In: Vasu T, Balasubramanian S, Kodivalasa M, Ingle PM. *Chronic Pain Management*, first edition. Shrewsbury: tfm Publishing Ltd; 2021, pp. 249–54.

Chapter 40

Harmful effects of opioids

Introduction

In treating chronic pain, opioids can become a problem, rather than be a solution. Although there are a range of very good opioid analgesics for the treatment of acute pain, evidence on their long-term use is limited. The Faculty of Pain Medicine's guideline 'Opioids Aware' explains that initiating, tapering or stopping opioid treatment should be made in agreement with the patient, their general practitioner and all members of the health care team involved in the patient's management. The same principles should apply to the management of chronic pain in patients with long COVID syndrome, with a cautious approach taken when prescribing opioids for these patients.

Opioid pharmacology

Opioid receptors are classified into four major types: mu (μ) opioid (MOP), kappa (κ) opioid (KOP), delta (δ) opioid (DOP) and nociceptin/orphanin FQ (N/OFQ). Opioid receptors are linked to inhibitory G-proteins and, on activation, close voltage-gated calcium channels, cause hyperpolarisation by potassium efflux and inhibit adenylyl cyclase, leading to decreased cyclic adenosine monophosphate (cAMP) and reduced release of neurotransmitters. Opioid medications inhibit the ascending excitatory pathway and activate the descending inhibitory pathway.

Common opioids

Morphine

Morphine has an oral bioavailability of 30% due to high first-pass metabolism. Given as an intravenous bolus, it has a peak action at 10 minutes. It is metabolised by glucuronidation in the liver and gut, and is excreted via the kidneys and in bile. Morphine-6-glucuronide can accumulate in liver failure. Side effects of morphine include respiratory depression, reduced response to carbon dioxide, suppression of cough response, hypotension, bradycardia, histamine release, sphincter of Oddi contraction and reduced levels of endocrine hormones (such as adrenocorticotrophic hormone), prolactin and gonadotrophic hormones.

Codeine

Codeine, or 3-methylmorphine, is a prodrug and a weak opioid. It is metabolised by glucuronidation. It undergoes N-demethylation to norcodeine. About 10% undergoes O-demethylation to morphine, with good analgesic effect, under the influence of cytochrome P450 enzyme (CYP2D6). CYP2D6 is absent in about 10% of Caucasians, in whom therefore codeine does not provide effective analgesia.

Oxycodone

Oxycodone is a MOP receptor agonist and a semi-synthetic derivative of thebaine. It has nearly twice the oral bioavailability of morphine. It is metabolised by N- and O-demethylation to noroxycodone and normorphine, respectively.

Tramadol

Tramadol is a racemic mixture of two stereoisomers. It works as a MOP receptor agonist, as well as reduces neuronal reuptake of serotonin. It has been found to be helpful in treating neuropathic pain. The National Institute for Health and Care Excellence (NICE) guidelines for the treatment of neuropathic pain recommend the addition of tramadol to other neuropathic pain medications. Tramadol is metabolised in the liver, and can interact with tricyclic antidepressants and selective serotonin reuptake inhibitors, causing serotonergic syndrome.

Fentanyl

Fentanyl is a selective MOP receptor agonist, with a rapid onset of action. It is 100 times more potent than morphine. Transdermal fentanyl is used in the treatment of chronic pain but has significant side effects at high doses, as is the case with the use of any opioid. Fentanyl has high solubility and is rapidly redistributed. Its side effects include chest wall rigidity and bronchospasm.

Buprenorphine

Buprenorphine is a semi-synthetic partial MOP agonist and a KOP antagonist. It also has agonist effects at the N/OFQ receptor. It is more potent than morphine and has a longer duration of action due to its high receptor affinity. It is commonly used as a transdermal preparation.

Common side effects

Common side effects of opioids include respiratory depression, constipation, drowsiness, confusion, nausea and tolerance. Of particular concern is physical dependence on opioids which is an important side effect of this drug class.

Warnings of long-term use of high-dose opioids

The evidence for opioid use in the long term, especially at high doses, is limited. Studies have reported significant harm and this has led to the creation of various guidelines to educate on the harms from opioid use. The Faculty of Pain Medicine of the Royal College of Anaesthetists has published the 'Opioids Aware' guideline to educate all health care professionals. The risk of harm from opioid use increases substantially at doses of above 120mg morphine equivalent per day, and help from a multidisciplinary team should be sought for at-risk patients.

Harm from long-term opioid use

Long-term opioid use at high doses causes endocrine and immunological problems, and reduces bone density. Further, long-term, high-dose opioid use can also lead to opioid-induced allodynia where opioids themselves can cause pain; this is due to changes in neuroplasticity at the opioid receptor level.

Harm specific to long COVID rehabilitation

Research has shown that high-dose opioid use over several months can suppress the immune system, which can worsen the prognosis for the acute phase of COVID-19, resulting in endothelial damage in the alveolar system and an increased risk of bacterial pneumonia. It is predicted that even after controlling for socio-economic factors, opioid misuse can lead to worse outcomes in patients with long COVID syndrome due to physiological and immunological effects of opioids.

In summary, it is prudent to avoid long-term use of opioids in patients with long COVID syndrome due to their associated risks. On the other hand, a short course of low-dose therapy can be used for pain relief, which will also help these patients participate in physiotherapy. It should be noted, however, that the evidence on long-term opioid use specifically in long COVID syndrome is very limited.

Key Points

- In treating chronic pain in patients with long COVID syndrome, opioids can become a problem, rather than be a solution.
- Long-term use of opioids at high doses can cause endocrine and immunological problems, as well as reduce bone density.
- Treatment with opioid doses of more than 120mg morphine equivalent per day requires specialist multidisciplinary input.

References

1.   Rajan RS, Ingle PM. Pharmacology — opioids. In: Vasu T, Balasubramanian S, Kodivalasa M, Ingle PM. *Chronic Pain Management*, first edition. Shrewsbury: tfm Publishing Ltd; 2021, pp. 235–44.

2.   Vasu T. Problems of opioid use in chronic pain. In: Vasu T, Balasubramanian S, Kodivalasa M, Ingle PM. *Chronic Pain Management*, first edition. Shrewsbury: tfm Publishing Ltd; 2021, pp. 245–8.

3.   National Institute for Health and Care Excellence (2013). Neuropathic pain in adults: pharmacological management in non-specialist settings. Clinical guideline [CG173]. Available from: https://www.nice.org.uk/guidance/cg173.

4.   Ataei M, Shirazi FM, Lamarine RJ, *et al.* A double-edged sword of using opioids and COVID-19: a toxicological view. *Substance Abuse Treatment, Prevention and Policy* 2020; 15: 91.

5.   Faculty of Pain Medicine. Opioids Aware. Available from: https://www.fpm.ac.uk/opioids-aware.

Section VI

Complementary therapies and pain clinic approach

Chapter 41

Acupuncture

Introduction

Complementary therapies have a role in the rehabilitation of patients with any chronic condition. The same principles apply to the management of patients with long COVID syndrome, with a multimodal and holistic approach to recovery. Acupuncture is one complementary intervention that has been found useful in the rehabilitation pathway in long COVID syndrome.

Mechanism of action

Patients with long COVID syndrome suffer from fatigue, weakness, muscle stiffness, neurological problems and chronic pain. Acupuncture can help in the management of these conditions, with the advantage of minimal side effects, compared with many other invasive medical interventions.

There is evidence of acupuncture being involved in the stimulation and neuromodulation of the nervous system. The technique stimulates the release of endorphins, activates inhibitory pathways, reduces activation of the pain matrix in the brain and modulates the pain pathway.

In the context of long COVID syndrome, acupuncture has been used to help relieve respiratory symptoms. Many long COVID patients with persistent respiratory problems have benefited from acupuncture as an adjuvant therapy.

Acupuncture can also be used to relieve stress, as well as various other related symptoms, especially given the increase in stress-related problems that have arisen due to the COVID pandemic.

Evidence base

It is too early to build an evidence base for the use of acupuncture in the management of long COVID syndrome, as is the case with other interventions. Currently, its use is based on extrapolation of evidence obtained in other chronic pain conditions, including from clinical practice and guidelines.

In the UK, the National Institute for Health and Care Excellence (NICE) does not recommend acupuncture in the treatment of mechanical low back pain. However, NICE recommends a course of ten sessions over 5–8 weeks for prophylactic treatment of chronic tension-type headaches. Acupuncture is a common intervention used to treat different types of pain, including widespread chronic pain, in most pain clinics in the UK.

A recent study based on bioinformatics and a network topology strategy showed that acupuncture can suppress inflammatory stress in COVID-19 illness. The study also showed that acupuncture activates neuroactive ligand-receptor interaction and the calcium signalling pathway, and may be beneficial to patients with COVID-19.

Case report on acupuncture use

A severe case of an elderly patient with COVID-19 from Wuhan, China, who recovered with the use of acupuncture and Chinese herbal medicine was recently reported in the literature. The authors reported that acupuncture significantly improved the patient's breathing function, increased SpO_2, decreased heart rate and improved blood markers for inflammation.

Guidance on acupuncture use in long COVID syndrome

A systematic review is under way to evaluate the effectiveness of acupuncture in patients with COVID-19, with analysis of chest computed tomography (CT) and nucleic acid detection of respiratory samples as primary outcomes and symptoms as secondary outcomes. The study group aims to provide evidence on whether acupuncture is effective in treating respiratory symptoms in patients affected by COVID-19, proposing that acupuncture may have a role in prevention, treatment and rehabilitation of patients with COVID-19.

The British Acupuncture Council has cited a number of studies showing the impact of acupuncture on the immune system and its anti-inflammatory effects. The Council proposes that acupuncture will prove very useful in treating COVID-19- and long COVID syndrome-related symptoms. According to the Council, acupuncture increases the body's ability to fight infections, while at the same time calming the occasional detrimental tendency of the body to overreact.

In summary, acupuncture can be a useful modality in the rehabilitation pathway for patients with long COVID syndrome. However, further research is needed to evaluate its specific benefits.

Key Points

- Acupuncture can be a useful intervention for patients with long COVID syndrome; it can help in the management of fatigue, pain, respiratory symptoms and stress.
- It has been suggested that acupuncture can modulate immune and inflammatory responses and could be beneficial in both the management of COVID-19 illness and rehabilitation of patients with long COVID syndrome.

References

1. Vasu T. Complementary therapies. In: Vasu T, Balasubramanian S, Kodivalasa M, Ingle PM. *Chronic Pain Management*, first edition. Shrewsbury: tfm Publishing Ltd; 2021, pp. 175–8.

2. Han Z, Zhang Y, Wang P, *et al*. Is acupuncture effective in the treatment of COVID-19 related symptoms? Based on bioinformatics/network topology strategy. *Brief Bioinform* 2021; bbab110.

3. Yin X, Cai S, Tao L, *et al*. Recovery of a patient with severe COVID-19 by acupuncture and Chinese herbal medicine adjuvant to standard care. *Journal of Integrative Medicine* 2021; 19: 460–6.

4. Chen Y, Zhu C, Xu Z, *et al*. Acupuncture for corona virus disease 2019. *Medicine* (Baltimore) 2020; 99: e22231.

5. British Acupuncture Council. COVID-19 FAQs. Available from: https://acupuncture.org.uk/safety-in-acupuncture/covid-19-faqs/.

Chapter 42

Transcutaneous electrical nerve stimulation

Introduction

Transcutaneous electrical nerve stimulation (TENS) is commonly used as part of many rehabilitation programmes and pain services in the management of chronic persistent pain. It can also be applied in patients with long COVID syndrome who have widespread or localised chronic pain.

Mechanism of action

TENS works on the principle of the gate control theory of pain. Stimulation of mechanoreceptors and A-beta nerve fibres block the transmission of pain signals via A-delta nerve fibres in the nociceptive pathway.

There is evidence that TENS stimulates the production of endorphins, the body's natural painkillers.

Evidence for use

TENS is one of the common modalities used as an adjuvant in multimodal therapy of chronic pain, despite limited evidence on its effectiveness in the management of chronic pain. TENS is used not only in neuromodulation therapy, but also to educate patients on the importance of supported self-management strategies. This education is vital to the recovery of patients from long COVID syndrome, as it is for patients with any other chronic condition.

Published studies on the use of TENS in COVID-19

A study published in November 2020 hypothesised that electrical stimulation improves respiratory function, reduces pain, boosts immunity and improves the efficacy of antiviral drugs in patients with COVID-19.

Practicalities of using TENS in long COVID syndrome

TENS is recommended for patients with long COVID syndrome for the following reasons, despite limited evidence on its use in this condition:

- It is non-invasive.
- It has a good safety profile, with few side effects.
- It is practical — its use is already established in other chronic conditions.
- It is easy to use — hence patients can self-manage.
- It is cheap.
- It is effective.
- It avoids the use of medications.
- It enjoys high satisfaction rates among its users.

TENS is a simple intervention that could be used as targeted therapy for musculoskeletal pain in patients with long COVID syndrome, along with other multimodal strategies.

Key Points

- TENS works on the principle of the gate control theory of pain.
- TENS can be part of a multimodal strategy in the rehabilitation of patients with long COVID syndrome, as well as in treating musculoskeletal pain in these patients.

References

1. Vasu T. Complementary therapies. In: Vasu T, Balasubramanian S, Kodivalasa M, Ingle PM. *Chronic Pain Management*, first edition. Shrewsbury: tfm Publishing Ltd; 2021, pp. 175–8.

2. Allawadhi P, Khurana A, Allwadhi S, *et al.* Potential of electric stimulation for the management of COVID-19. *Med Hypotheses* 2020; 144: 110259.

Chapter 43

Psychology

Introduction

Strategies for managing mental health and mood problems in patients with long COVID syndrome are elaborated in Chapter 32. Recently, there have been huge controversies over the role of psychology in the management of long COVID syndrome, as well as much debate on the subject. This chapter will discuss in detail the role of psychology in managing this condition and the controversies over psychological interventions.

NICE guideline on long COVID syndrome

The National Institute for Health and Care Excellence (NICE) guideline on long COVID syndrome has made clear recommendations on the use of multidisciplinary rehabilitation services, including physical, psychological and psychiatric input.

Controversies over the role of psychology

The role of psychology in the rehabilitation of patients with chronic conditions is well established and psychological interventions have been used as a standard of care for many decades. Given the emotional and psychological sequelae of COVID-19 illness, the pandemic, social isolation and persistent symptoms in long COVID syndrome, it is natural that patients will need psychological help as part of their comprehensive multimodal rehabilitation care package.

Post-traumatic stress, hospital stay, intensive care-related sequelae, sleep problems, loss of relatives and/or close friends, nightmares and delirium following acute illness are but a few typical reasons highlighting the need for psychological therapies in patients with long COVID syndrome, in whom the role of such interventions is well established and proven.

However, some patient groups and associations, including the ME Association, have raised concerns about the role of psychological therapies, such as cognitive behavioural therapy (CBT), in managing patients with long COVID syndrome. They argue that sole reliance on a physical approach, such as the use of graded exercise therapy, and psychological interventions, such as CBT, might mean that patients do not undergo proper assessments or receive appropriate symptomatic treatment. Some also argue that the use of psychological interventions is based on poor-quality evidence showing marginal short-term improvements. In the UK, in response to these concerns, NICE has cautioned against graded exercise therapy, while further updates on its guidance are awaited.

NICE guidance recognises both the physical and psychological impact of long COVID syndrome on affected individuals. However, the British Psychological Society has expressed its disappointment and dissatisfaction that the guidance lacks detailed recommendations regarding multidisciplinary rehabilitation and is completely silent on what this rehabilitation should consist of and how the rehabilitation pathway should be set up.

Yellow flags

As in any chronic illness, it is a routine practice for rehabilitation teams to assess for the presence of yellow flags in patients. These are psychological factors that are indicative of long-term chronicity and disability.

Yellow flags include: a negative belief that their condition is harmful and disabling; fear-avoidance behaviour and activity restrictions; expectation of passive treatments, rather than the patient taking control of their management; a tendency for depression and social withdrawal; and social or financial problems.

It is important to address these issues right at the beginning of the rehabilitation pathway, so appropriate care is given and appropriate actions taken to prevent chronicity. Addressing these issues, however, is more difficult in long COVID syndrome, given this illness has devastating effects on social, financial and psychological aspects of patients' lives.

Cognitive behavioural therapy

CBT has been found effective in providing patients with coping strategies. CBT helps to manage mental illness by changing the way a patient thinks (cognition) and behaves (behaviour), so they can change the way they feel.

Thoughts, feelings and actions are interrelated, and negative thinking can result in a patient being caught in a vicious cycle. The role of CBT is to explore these interlinks and address the problem by changing the patient's negative thinking pattern. It helps the patient break down the problem of long COVID syndrome into smaller chunks, so they gain confidence in dealing and coping with the problem in a positive way.

CBT aims to identify challenging, unhelpful thoughts in patients with long COVID syndrome. Once identified, the patient is taken through graded exposure, thereby reducing unhelpful behaviours and removing unnecessary fears.

Acceptance and commitment therapy

While CBT teaches patients how to control their thoughts, feelings and memories, acceptance and commitment therapy (ACT) involves the patient accepting and embracing their problem and committing to their recovery from these difficulties. ACT is based on the relational frame theory which proposes that rational skills may not be effective when faced with a psychological problem, and teaches the patient to accept the problem as normal and learn ways to live more healthily. It uses mindfulness-based approaches which are discussed below. The use of metaphors is common in ACT to engage the patient in the acceptance pathway.

ACT focuses on the patient embracing their thoughts and feelings, leading to commitment to recovery and behavioural change. Although it may not necessarily help the patient to accept the sequelae of long COVID syndrome, it will help them to accept the unwanted experiences suffered as a consequence of the condition.

The six core principles of ACT that help to develop psychological flexibility include:

- Cognitive defusion.
- Acceptance.
- Being in the present moment.
- Self as context.
- Discovering values.
- Committed action.

Mindfulness-based approaches

Mindfulness focuses on the present moment, rather than dwelling on multiple problems and catastrophising. It helps the patient to be fully aware of where they are and what they are doing, and not to be overwhelmed by what happens outside.

It uses meditation techniques that help the patient live in, and concentrate on, the present moment, using any of the senses, including touch, sight, sound, taste or smell. Thus, mindfulness creates awareness of thoughts in the present moment.

Mindfulness-based stress reduction and mindfulness-based cognitive therapy may have a significant role in the rehabilitation pathway for patients with long COVID syndrome, if incorporated as part of multimodal treatment.

Approach to psychology

We need to be aware of the controversies over various therapies in long COVID syndrome, so we can understand the limitations of these interventions and select appropriate treatment pathways. It will take some time before high-quality research evidence is available in this domain. However, it is clear that long COVID syndrome affects the emotional state of patients, as well as their quality of life.

The behavioural patterns and coping styles of sufferers of long COVID syndrome can determine their functional outcomes and quality of life. It is therefore important to include multidisciplinary assessment and treatment at the earliest opportunity in the rehabilitation pathway for patients with long COVID syndrome.

Key Points

- As recommended by NICE, it is important to assess for psychological and psychiatric problems in patients with long COVID syndrome, and not only for physical problems.
- There are controversies over the use of graded exercise therapy and CBT in patients with long COVID syndrome and it is important to understand these concerns.
- Management of patients with long COVID syndrome should include assessing their specific treatment needs and offering psychological help as part of the multimodal rehabilitation pathway.

References

1. Vasu T. Psychology in chronic pain. In: Vasu T, Balasubramanian S, Kodivalasa M, Ingle PM. *Chronic Pain Management*, first edition. Shrewsbury: tfm Publishing Ltd; 2021, pp. 183–8.

2. National Institute for Health and Care Excellence (2020). COVID-19 rapid guideline: managing the long-term effects of COVID-19. NICE guideline [NG188]. Available from: https://www.nice.org.uk/guidance/ng188.

3. ME Association (2021). BMJ rapid response Re: ME/CFS and long COVID: moving beyond the controversy — by Dr Charles Shepherd. Available from: https://meassociation.org.uk/2021/06/bmj-response-moving-beyond-the-controversy-by-dr-charles-shepherd/.

4. The British Psychological Society (2020). BPS responds to new NICE guidance on managing the long-term effects of Covid-19. Available from: https://www.bps.org.uk/news-and-policy/bps-responds-new-nice-guidance-managing-long-term-effects-covid-19.

5. Torjesen I. NICE cautions against using graded exercise therapy for patients recovering from covid-19. *BMJ* 2020; 370: m2912.

Chapter 44

Pain clinic approach

Introduction

Rehabilitation pathways in long COVID syndrome vary, depending on the presenting symptoms and their severity (see Chapter 23 for details on the pathways). However, some patients may have a pain-predominant presentation, weeks or months after having had COVID-19 illness, and may need referral to chronic pain services. This chapter will elaborate in detail the structured approach in the management of these patients.

Need for pain clinic referral

Long COVID syndrome is considered to represent another 'wave of the pandemic' that will be a long-term burden on health care provision and society. The majority of patients with long COVID syndrome will be managed in the community with a supported self-management approach and advice (see Chapter 23). Of those needing specialist support, not all will be referred to a specialist assessment centre due to financial constraints in the health care system. Therefore, general practitioners should use a structured approach when assessing patients and make referrals for specialist support based on their clinical presentation and needs.

Chronic pain clinic services have huge expertise in setting up rehabilitation pathways for pain patients (most of which are discussed in this book). It is important that health care policymakers should allocate appropriate funding for the provision of chronic pain services.

The biopsychosocial model

Most chronic pain services use the biopsychosocial model in patient rehabilitation (see Chapter 27). Even though pain is the predominant symptom, expert pain clinicians recognise the role of psychological and social factors and use a multidisciplinary, multimodal approach to management that will help improve patients' quality of life.

Structured approach

Pain clinic services use a structured approach when managing patients. Most services require patients to complete an assessment questionnaire before the first appointment to determine the overall impact of pain on their life. Assessment questionnaires may vary across services but they always include questions assessing the psychological and social aspects of the pain problem. Some services also use specific psychological and disability questionnaires, with many focusing on anxiety and depression scores.

In clinic consultations, elaborate history taking is key to engaging patients in their management, while also reassuring them that they are being listened to by the clinician, particularly as many patients feel that their complaints were not always listened to properly in the past. Listening is an active form of communication and an art in health care.

A detailed physical examination (general as well as focused based on affected body areas) is part of the pain clinic consultation. This will then enable the clinician to generate a differential diagnosis and discuss this with their patient. Appropriate investigations can then be arranged, and a comprehensive multimodal treatment plan set.

Patient education is key when setting a comprehensive pain management plan, where detailed discussions with the patient on their condition and treatment plans will help them to engage in the recovery pathway.

Management plans offered in pain clinics

Pain clinics always follow a multimodal treatment approach:

- Patient education is the most crucial part of the treatment plan.
- Physiotherapy forms the basis for recovery with exercises for core muscle strengthening and general posture and focused exercises. Pacing strategies are vital in any rehabilitation plan.
- Complementary therapies include acupuncture, transcutaneous electrical nerve stimulation (TENS) and various other therapies based on availability and expertise.
- Medications include analgesics, neuropathic drugs, topical agents and other medications/adjuvants.
- Injections include various injections based on local pathology or generalised infusion therapies.
- Psychological assessment and therapies.
- Group rehabilitation programmes.

Some pain services use other interventions, including, but not limited to occupational therapy, relaxation and distraction therapies, neuromodulatory procedures, such as spinal cord or peripheral nerve stimulation, and intrathecal implantable device interventions.

Specialised pain interventions in long COVID syndrome

In addition to the common interventions listed above, specific interventions are also used in patients with long COVID syndrome, including intravenous lidocaine infusion, intramuscular injection of botulinum toxin, pulsed radiofrequency neuromodulation and other newer neuromodulatory techniques. These will be discussed in Chapters 45, 46 and 47.

Outcomes and evaluation

Most pain clinic services use some form of patient-reported outcome measures (PROMs) to assess the quality of care provided to their patients from their perspective. Clinical audits and clinical governance are fundamental to the evaluation of outcomes and assessing for any necessary changes to current services.

Communication with other teams

There is direct liaison between pain clinic teams and patients' general practitioners to make sure that the comprehensive plan set by the pain clinic is followed in the community. In many circumstances, the general practitioner will be the sole drug prescriber, in particular of opioids and stronger analgesics, to avoid the harm of medications.

For patients who are also under the care of other services, including specialist long COVID clinics, it is important that pain clinicians liaise with these other specialist teams to ensure a properly structured rehabilitation pathway.

Role of the patient

Along the recovery pathway, patients will be at the centre of their comprehensive treatment plan. Any intervention will be focused on the patients themselves that will allow them to take control of their own management. Therefore, patients should be fully educated and encouraged to take charge of their own recovery/rehabilitation plan.

As mentioned before, supported self-management is the key to patient recovery from long COVID syndrome and this approach should be encouraged in the pain clinic also.

Key Points

- Long COVID patients whose predominant symptom is pain will benefit from referral to chronic pain services.
- Chronic pain services have huge expertise that are beneficial to patient rehabilitation.
- Pain clinics use a structured approach to help long COVID patients who present with pain.
- A comprehensive multimodal biopsychosocial plan is used by pain clinic services to help in the recovery of long COVID patients.

References

1. Vasu T. The biopsychosocial model. In: Vasu T, Balasubramanian S, Kodivalasa M, Ingle PM. *Chronic Pain Management*, first edition. Shrewsbury: tfm Publishing Ltd; 2021, pp. 21–4.

Section VII

Novel pain therapies in long COVID syndrome

Chapter 45

Intravenous lidocaine infusion

Introduction

Various treatments are being tested in the management of long COVID patients who suffer from chronic pain. A novel treatment that holds promise is intravenous lidocaine infusion. The use of an intravenous lidocaine infusion is well established in the treatment of chronic pain conditions such as fibromyalgia, albeit with limited evidence, and many pain clinics offer this as part of standard treatment in fibromyalgia. Another use of an intravenous lidocaine bolus is in anaesthesia and intensive care practice to attenuate the stress response during laryngoscopy.

Lidocaine is a local anaesthetic that, when given intravenously at high doses, can cause neuromodulation and help in widespread pain relief. The role of lidocaine in COVID-19 illness has been studied, and its use in patients with COVID-19 has been based on evidence extrapolated from non-COVID-related studies. This chapter will discuss the practicalities and usefulness of this technique in the context of treating long COVID syndrome.

Mechanism of action

Neutrophils play a major role in infections and can influence the development of organ damage as well as the risk of mortality. In sepsis, phagocytosis and oxidative burst reactions induce the release of neutrophil extracellular traps (NETs), which are web-like structures composed of deoxyribonucleic acid (DNA) that are studded with proteins and help in trapping pathogenic organisms. The process of NET formation is known as NETosis. Dysregulation of NETosis causes collateral damage and affects the pulmonary, cardiovascular and renal systems. NETs have a role in cytokine storm and hypercoagulability, both of which have been proposed to be responsible for high morbidity and mortality in COVID-19 illness.

The process of NETosis involves two mediators: high mobility group box-1 (HMGB-1) and granulocyte colony-stimulating factor (G-CSF). Lidocaine can inhibit both HBGB-1 and G-CSF, leading to reduced NETosis, and thereby preventing or reducing the cytokine storm and associated morbidity.

Citrullinated histone H3 (Cit-H3) is a specific biomarker for NETs and high levels of Cit-H3 have been observed in COVID-19 patients. Studies have proposed NETs as a prognostic indicator of venous thromboembolism.

Other supporting evidence for the use of lidocaine in COVID-19

Other evidence supporting the use of lidocaine in COVID-19 patients includes the following:

- Lidocaine has possible anti-inflammatory actions.
- It may reduce the severity of the cytokine storm.
- It is used in chronic pain conditions.
- It is used intraoperatively in patients undergoing major surgeries, as well as in those undergoing laryngoscopy, to reduce the stress response.
- It has cytoprotective effects.
- It can delay ischaemic changes.
- It has direct spasmolytic effects.
- It has an ion channel-blocking effect.
- It is a repolarising agent.

A systematic review published in March 2020 showed that the perioperative use of intravenous lidocaine led to large reductions in post-extubation cough (number needed to treat = 5) and postoperative sore throat (number needed to treat = 4), with no increased risk of harm. Among proposed mechanisms of action is suppression of the airway's excitatory sensory C fibres and release of sensory neuropeptides.

Previous research has shown that intravenous lidocaine reduces endotoxin release and cytokine surge in acute lung injury.

Other studies have also examined the use of nebulised lidocaine as a possible treatment against respiratory illness caused by severe acute respiratory syndrome coronavirus 2 (SARS-CoV-2), due to the anti-inflammatory effects of lidocaine.

The effects of lidocaine mentioned above are not specifically proven in COVID-19 illness. Existing scientific theories propose these as causes of morbidity in COVID-19 and lidocaine can be used to reduce the damage caused by the viral illness.

The role of lidocaine in pain relief in long COVID syndrome

Given the possibility of persistent low-grade inflammation in long COVID syndrome, intravenous lidocaine can be used to manage systemic symptoms, in addition to its pain-relieving actions. Intravenous lidocaine is used by pain clinicians to treat patients with widespread chronic pain conditions, and can be used also in those with long COVID syndrome since these patients present with similar pain patterns. The use of intravenous lidocaine can break the vicious cycle of pain and therefore help patients to engage in their pain management, without using other pharmacological agents, thereby minimising the risk of drug side effects.

Dosages and side effects of intravenous lidocaine

Standard textbooks have quoted using intravenous lidocaine at doses of 3–5mg/kg body weight over 30–60 minutes. Side effects include: arrhythmias, blood pressure changes, nausea/vomiting, numbness and tingling, dizziness, headache, toxicity and seizures.

Key Points

- Intravenous lidocaine is a common intervention used in the treatment of chronic widespread pain.
- Lidocaine reduces the formation of NETs, thereby reducing the severity of the cytokine storm; this will improve the outcomes of COVID-19.
- Intravenous lidocaine can be beneficial to long COVID patients who suffer from chronic pain.

References

1. Balasubramanian S. Infusion therapies in chronic pain management. In: Vasu T, Balasubramanian S, Kodivalasa M, Ingle PM. *Chronic Pain Management*, first edition. Shrewsbury: tfm Publishing Ltd; 2021, pp. 161–4.

2. Finnerty DT, Buggy DJ. A novel role for lidocaine in COVID-19 patients? *Br J Anaesth* 2020; 125: E391–4.

3. Tadie J, Bao H, Jiang S, *et al*. HMGB1 promotes neutrophil extracellular trap formation through interactions with toll-like receptor 4. *Am J Physiol Lung Cell Mol Physiol* 2013; 304: L342–9.

4. Wang H, Liu Y, Yan H, *et al*. Intraoperative systemic lidocaine inhibits the expression of HMGB1 in patients undergoing radical hysterectomy. *Int J Clin Exp Med* 2014; 7: 3398–403.

5. D'Agostino G, Saporito A, Cecchinato V, *et al*. Lidocaine inhibits cytoskeletal remodelling and human breast cancer cell migration. *Br J Anaesth* 2018; 121: 962–8.

6. Snoderly HT, Boone BA, Bennewitz MF. Neutrophil extracellular traps in breast cancer and beyond: current perspectives on NET stimuli, thrombosis and metastasis, and clinical utility for diagnosis and treatment. *Breast Cancer Res* 2019; 21: 145.

7. Galos EV, Tat T, Popa R, *et al*. Neutrophil extracellular trapping and angiogenesis biomarkers after intravenous or inhalation anaesthesia with or without intravenous lidocaine for breast cancer surgery: a prospective, randomised trial. *Br J Anaesth* 2020; 125: 712–21.

8. Hollmann MW, Durieux ME, Fisher DM. Local anesthetics and the inflammatory response: a new therapeutic indication? *Anesthesiology* 2000; 93: 858–75.

9. Yang SS, Wang NN, Postonogova T, *et al*. Intravenous lidocaine to prevent postoperative airway complications in adults: a systematic review and meta-analysis. *Br J Anaesth* 2020; 124: 314–23.

10. Mikawa K, Maekawa N, Nishina K, *et al*. Effect of lidocaine pretreatment on endotoxin-induced lung injury in rabbits. *Anesthesiology* 1994; 81: 689–99.

11. Malik NA, Hammodi A, Jaiswara DR. Lignocaine's substantial role in COVID-19 management: potential remedial and therapeutic implications. *Anaesth Pain Intensive Care* 2020; 24: 59–63.

Chapter 46

Nerve blocks

Introduction

Nerve blocks are common interventions used in the rehabilitation of patients with chronic pain conditions. They help to break the vicious cycle of pain, encourage patients and give them the confidence they need so they can engage in physiotherapy and their supported self-management pathway. The same principle applies to the treatment of patients with long COVID syndrome who suffer from chronic pain. Many pain services use either local or central neuraxial nerve blocks in the rehabilitation of long COVID patients.

The role of regional anaesthesia and nerve blocks

Throughout the COVID-19 pandemic, the use of regional anaesthesia has been recommended, wherever possible, for anaesthetic/analgesic indications to minimise the risk of generating aerosols from general anaesthetics. Nerve blocks have been commonly used throughout the pandemic for various indications.

The use of nerve blocks by chronic pain services can be beneficial to long COVID patients with chronic pain by helping them to engage in their recovery pathway.

Common injections used by pain services for long COVID syndrome

Trigger point injections with ultrasound guidance are commonly used in rehabilitation programmes for localised pain relief. Engagement in physiotherapy is vital to post-injection care. Advice on exercise, pacing strategies and the need to keep active should be given to the patient in order to help break the pain cycle.

Peripheral nerve blocks, such as suprascapular and greater occipital nerve blocks, mechanical spinal injections and other injections, can be easily incorporated into rehabilitation programmes. Chronic pain services offer huge expertise in performing peripheral nerve blocks on an outpatient basis in a cost-effective and clinically safe way.

Avoiding steroid use in long COVID syndrome

The use of steroids should be avoided, or at least minimised, in patients with long COVID syndrome due to the risk of immunosuppression and resultant infection. Steroids also have many side effects, especially at high doses, including reduced bone density, hormone problems, menorrhagia and cataracts. Pulsed radiofrequency neuromodulation and radiofrequency denervation are preferred alternatives, especially given the availability of these techniques in many pain services, and their good safety profile and ease of application.

Clinical guidance on the use of steroids in the context of COVID-19, published jointly by various medical societies, recommends that alternatives to steroids should always be considered, and if not possible, the lowest possible steroid dose should be used for the shortest possible time, in which case the benefits of using steroids should outweigh the risks. Even in epidural or targeted nerve root blocks for severe radiculopathy, the guidance recommends the use of local anaesthetics only or the lowest possible steroid dose.

Guidance from the British Society of Skeletal Radiologists also emphasises the need to avoid steroid injections, whenever possible, in articular spaces, soft tissues and perineural areas, during the COVID-19 pandemic. Non-steroidal pain injections are suggested instead as an alternative.

The College of Podiatry and the Faculty of Podiatric Medicine of the Royal College of Physicians and Surgeons of Glasgow have also cautioned against the use of corticosteroids and advised clinicians to first explore all possible non-injection alternatives for pain management.

Key Points

- **Nerve injections can help patients with long COVID syndrome to engage in their physiotherapy.**
- **It is advisable to avoid steroids or to assess the risks and benefits before the use of steroid injections.**

References

1. Balasubramanian S. Infusion therapies in chronic pain management. In: Vasu T, Balasubramanian S, Kodivalasa M, Ingle PM. *Chronic Pain Management*, first edition. Shrewsbury: tfm Publishing Ltd; 2021, pp. 161–4.

2. British Society for Rheumatology (2020). Clinical guide during the COVID-19 pandemic for the management of patients with musculoskeletal and rheumatic conditions. Available from: https://www.rheumatology.org.uk/Portals/0/Documents/COVID-19/MSK_rheumatology_corticosteroid_guidance.pdf.

3. Fuscia D, Dalili D, Rennie W, et al. (2020). Recommendations of the British Society of Skeletal Radiologists. The safety of corticosteroid injections during the COVID-19 global pandemic. Available from: https://www.wnswphn.org.au/uploads/documents/Resources/Coronavirus/Musculoskeletal_Radiology_during_the_COVID-19_Global_Pandemic.pdf.

4. The College of Podiatry, the Faculty of Podiatric Medicine of the Royal College of Physicians and Surgeons of Glasgow (2020). Steroid injections and COVID-19 — updated guidance. Available from: https://news.rcpsg.ac.uk/news/steroid-injections-and-covid-19-updated-guidance-november-2020/.

Chapter 47

Botox treatment for headache

Introduction

Headache can be a troublesome symptom in long COVID syndrome. Similarly to other chronic headache conditions, complementary therapies, such as acupuncture, relaxation and breathing exercises, can help long COVID patients suffering from headaches. Pain services also use techniques such as trigger point injections into muscles and greater occipital nerve blocks to treat headaches. In persistent pain, there is a role for botulinum toxin in the treatment of chronic headaches.

The impact of the COVID pandemic on patients with headaches

A web-based survey showed that, compared to the pre-COVID pandemic period, 59.6% of patients with headaches reported an increase in migraine frequency, 64.1% reported an increase in severity and 58.7% reported overuse of analgesic medications. Of those who had COVID-19, 63.4% reported worsening of their headaches. Therefore, the COVID pandemic has had an overall negative impact on patients with migraine.

Botulinum toxin and its use

Botulinum toxin is extracted from the anaerobic bacteria *Clostridium botulinum*, with seven of its 40 subtypes showing antigen specificity. The toxin is organised as a double-chain protein, with the light chain being the active form. Botulinum toxin type A (BoNT-A) and type B (BoNT-B) are commonly used in the practice of pain medicine.

Mechanism of action of botulinum toxin

At the neuromuscular junction, a complex of soluble N-ethylmaleimide-sensitive factor attachment protein receptor (SNARE) proteins, including syntaxin, synaptobrevin and synaptosomal-associated protein 25 (SNAP-25), are involved in the release of acetylcholine, resulting in muscle contraction. Botulinum toxin blocks the presynaptic release of acetylcholine at the neuromuscular junction by breaking down this SNARE protein complex, causing muscle relaxation which leads to its analgesic effects. This process also releases neuropeptides such as substance P and calcitonin gene-related peptide (CGRP) in nociceptive neurons, contributing to analgesia.

The current evidence and guidance on the use of Botox® as headache treatment

The PREEMPT (Phase 3 REsearch Evaluating Migraine Prophylaxis Therapy) trial showed that onabotulinum toxin A (Botox®) is an effective prophylactic treatment for chronic headache, improves headache symptoms and reduces headache-related disability, with improved functioning and quality of life.

The National Institute for Health and Care Excellence (NICE) in its technology appraisal guidance has recommended BoNT-A for chronic migraine prophylaxis in patients suffering from headaches for at least 15 days every month and who have not responded to at least three medications. If patients show improved headache symptoms, BoNT-A can be continued. However, it should be discontinued if patients show less than 30% symptomatic relief after two injections.

Usage practicalities

As per the NICE guidelines, Botox® is injected in 31 sites or more, at a dose of 5 units for each site, with a maximum of 200 units.

For long COVID patients presenting with resistant headaches unresponsive to other simple treatments, Botox® can be used.

Botox® and the COVID-19 vaccine

According to the American Migraine Foundation, there is speculation that the COVID-19 vaccine can make Botox® less effective, although there is no direct evidence. The Foundation recommends to prioritise vaccination in migraine sufferers and to leave a 2-week interval between receiving the COVID-19 vaccine and Botox® injections.

Key Points

- Botulinum toxin blocks the presynaptic release of acetylcholine at the neuromuscular junction; it breaks down the SNARE protein complex and prevents release of the neurotransmitter.
- NICE recommends Botox® for patients whose headaches last for more than 15 days every month and who have not responded to three different medications.

References

1. Kodivalasa M. Pharmacology of other medications. In: Vasu T, Balasubramanian S, Kodivalasa M, Ingle PM. *Chronic Pain Management*, first edition. Shrewsbury: tfm Publishing Ltd; 2021, pp. 285–8.

2. Al-Hashel JY, Ismail II. Impact of coronavirus disease 2019 (COVID-19) pandemic on patients with migraine: a web-based survey study. *J Headache Pain* 2020; 21: 115.

3. Dodick DW, Turkel CC, DeGryse RE, *et al.* OnabotulinumtoxinA for treatment of chronic migraine: pooled results from the double-blind, randomised, placebo-controlled phases of the PREEMPT clinical program. *Headache* 2010; 50: 921–36.

4. National Institute for Health and Care Excellence (2012). Botulinium toxin type A for the prevention of headaches in adults with chronic migraine. Technology appraisal guidance [TA260]. Available from: https://www.nice.org.uk/guidance/ta260.

5. American Migraine Foundation (2021). Questions about the COVID-19 vaccines for people living with migraine. Available from: https://americanmigrainefoundation.org/resource-library/questions-about-the-covid-19-vaccines-for-people-living-with-migraine/.

Section VIII

Long COVID in children

Chapter 48

Long COVID syndrome in children

Introduction

In June 2021, the NHS in the UK announced plans to offer specialist long COVID services for children and young people. A total of 15 new paediatric hubs drawing expertise from different specialties were set up to help young children with long COVID syndrome, as well as their families.

Prevalence of long COVID syndrome in children

The majority of children and young people recover from COVID-19 illness. However, based on a survey by the Office for National Statistics, 7.4% of children aged 2–11 years and 8.2% of those aged 12–16 years suffer from long COVID syndrome.

A prospective cohort study published in *The Lancet* in 2021 on school-aged children in the UK reported that only 1.8% of children experienced long COVID-related symptoms for more than 8 weeks and 4.4% had persistent illness for more than 4 weeks. The limitation of this study was the use of a mobile application (app) for self-reporting and therefore, potentially many patients could have been missed with lack of motivation to use the app.

An Italian study reported that 58.2% of children with COVID-19 illness had persistent symptoms even at a median of 162 days after initial diagnosis, with 35.7% having one or two symptoms and 22.5% three or more symptoms. Insomnia was common, with 23.3% of children affected 60–120 days after the initial diagnosis and 16.2% after 120 days. Persistent muscle pain was observed in 6.7% of children after 60–120 days and in 8.8% after 120 days. Headache was persistent in 23.3% of children after 60–120 days and in 7.4% after 120 days.

A European prospective study found an incidence of 24.3% of children aged less than 18 years with long COVID symptoms, even at more than 5 months after COVID-19 illness. One in ten of affected children reported multisystemic problems due to long COVID syndrome.

An Australian study also reported a high incidence of long COVID syndrome in children, with 8% of children remaining symptomatic after 3–6 months of COVID-19 illness.

It is essential to gather further epidemiological data, while avoiding any bias, to determine with more accuracy the incidence of long COVID syndrome in children.

Symptoms of long COVID syndrome in children

Common symptoms of long COVID syndrome in children include mild persistent cough, fatigue, sleep disturbance and sensory problems.

Apart from long COVID symptoms, children have also been subjected to social and psychological effects of lockdown and isolation, as well as restricted education and social interactions, all of which have a potentially lifelong impact on their development and mental well-being.

Risk factors for long COVID syndrome in children

Long COVID syndrome has been found to be more common in older-aged children (6–11 years; odds ratio of 2.74) and those with a history of allergic disease (odds ratio of 1.67).

Management

Management principles for treating long COVID syndrome in children are similar to those used in the rehabilitation pathway for adults. Unfortunately, the availability of long COVID specialist clinics, specialist expertise and access to rehabilitation services are significantly limited in many countries. Chronic pain services would be beneficial to children with long COVID syndrome who suffer persistent pain. These services have the specialist skills and expertise required to set up a focused plan with supported self-management and is based on a multidisciplinary, multimodal biopsychosocial model.

Key Points

- The NHS in the UK has recognised the need for support provision to children with long COVID syndrome and has since established 15 paediatric hubs.
- Various incidence rates of long COVID syndrome in children have been reported, so further epidemiological data are needed, while avoiding bias.
- Any social and psychological effects as a result of lockdown due to the COVID-19 pandemic can have a potentially lifelong impact on child development.

References

1.   National Health Service (2021). NHS sets up specialist young people's services in £100 million long COVID care expansion. Available from: https://www.england.nhs.uk/2021/06/nhs-sets-up-specialist-young-peoples-services-in-100-million-long-covid-care-expansion/.

2.   Molteni E, Sudre CH, Canas LS, *et al*. Illness duration and symptom profile in symptomatic UK school-aged children tested for SARS-CoV-2. *Lancet Child Adolesc Health* 2021; 5: 708–18.

3.   Buonsenso D, Munblit D, De Rose C, *et al*. Preliminary evidence on long COVID in children. *Acta Paediatr* 2021; 110: 2208–11.

4.   Osmanov IM, Spiridonova E, Bobkova P, *et al*. Risk factors for long COVID in previously hospitalised children using the ISARIC global follow-up protocol: a prospective cohort study. *Eur Respir J* 2021; in press. https://doi.org/10.1183/13993003.01341-2021.

5.   Say D, Crawford N, McNab S, *et al*. Post-acute COVID-19 outcomes in children with mild and asymptomatic disease. *Lancet Child Adolesc Health* 2021; 5: E22–3.

Section IX

Patient support groups for long COVID syndrome

Chapter 49

Patient support groups for long COVID syndrome

Introduction

Long COVID syndrome is a relatively new condition with many complex presentations. Health care professionals may not be aware of all the various presentations and often the condition can be very challenging to manage. Leadership, political willingness and financial resources are needed to create pathways for the specialist rehabilitation and treatment of long COVID syndrome. Under a financially constrained health care system, setting up such specialist services can be difficult without patient group lobbying. Liaison among patient groups, the Government, health care delivery systems and other stakeholders helps to ensure that patients' voices are heard and treatment strategies are based on their needs and wishes.

LongCovidSOS

The LongCovidSOS campaign was formed as a result of patients suffering from long COVID syndrome not being heard by health care professionals and the Government in terms of their COVID-related suffering and problems. The aim of the campaign is to put pressure on the Government to recognise long COVID patients' needs and to raise awareness among the public and employers. One such example is the launching of the 'Message in a Bottle' campaign, the aim of which can be summarised as 'Recognition Research Rehab'.

In July 2020, an open letter to political and managerial leaders was published that included more than 1000 signatures, demanding the setting up of a working group to investigate long COVID syndrome and the commissioning of urgent research into the condition.

Long COVID Support

Long COVID Support is a peer support and advocacy group for people living with long COVID syndrome. The charity group has helped by questioning whether health care policies are beneficial to patients suffering from long COVID syndrome and has written letters to ministers lobbying on behalf of long COVID patients.

Long COVID Wales

Long COVID Wales is a devolved Welsh campaign set up by more than 42,000 Welsh patients. The group raises awareness of long COVID syndrome via social media platforms such as Twitter and Facebook.

Long COVID Scotland

Long COVID Scotland collaborates with partners to find solutions for people living with long COVID syndrome. It has more than 40,000 members.

Patient-Led Research Collaborative on long COVID syndrome

This is a self-organised group of long COVID patients working on patient-led research on the long COVID experience. They have published surveys focused on patients' long COVID experience.

Body Politic COVID-19 Support Group

Through a global network of COVID-19 patients, chronic illness allies and health and disability advocates, this support group aims to promote patient-driven whole-person care and well-being. It has more than 11,000 members.

Other long COVID patient experience and support groups

The British Association for Performing Arts Medicine (BAPAM), via blogs, link to support groups so patient experience, advice and resources can be shared. As the experience of suffering from long COVID syndrome can be isolating, sharing experiences among other long COVID sufferers can be invaluable.

Key Points

- The aim of patient groups is to lobby and liaise with the Government, health care managers and other stakeholders to raise awareness of long COVID syndrome and ensure patients' voices are heard.
- Making patients' voices heard ensures that interventions are targeted and specific to patients' needs and wishes.

References

1.   LongCovidSOS. Available from: https://www.longcovidsos.org.
2.   Long Covid Support. Available from: https://www.longcovid.org.
3.   Long Covid Wales. Available from: https://twitter.com/LongCovidWales.
4.   Long Covid Scotland. Available from: https://www.longcovid.scot.

5.   Patient-Led Research Collaborative. Available from: https://patientresearchcovid19.com/.

6.   Body Politic Covid-19 Support Group. Available from: https://www.wearebodypolitic.com/covid19.

7.   British Association for Performing Arts Medicine (2021). Long COVID: patient experience and support groups. Available from: https://www.bapam.org.uk/long-covid-patient-experience-and-support-groups/.

Section X

New research interventions

Chapter 50

Research on long COVID syndrome

Introduction

Long COVID syndrome is a new condition that needs to be researched well in order to build up an evidence base that will help to streamline treatment and rehabilitation pathways. In the meantime, management of this condition continues to rely on extrapolation from general rehabilitation principles until sufficient research data on long COVID syndrome will be available from randomised double-blind trials in the future.

Government initiatives in the United Kingdom

In the UK, in July 2021, the Government announced the allocation of nearly £20 million through the National Institute for Health Research (NIHR) to set up 15 new studies to investigate the diagnosis and treatment of long COVID syndrome. Over £50 million has also been invested by the UK government in long COVID research for better understanding of this long-term condition. Some of the projects include:

- STIMULATE-ICP (Symptoms, Trajectory, Inequalities and Management: Understanding Long-COVID to Address and Transform Existing Integrated Care Pathways), University College London: involves more than 4500 participants (awarded about £7 million).

This study assesses treatment efficacy after 3 months, mental health and outcomes. Magnetic resonance imaging is used to assess for potential organ damage. Rehabilitation is enhanced with a special app.

- Cardiff University Immunologic study: a study awarded £800,000 to investigate immunologic and virologic determinants of long COVID syndrome.
- ReDIRECT, University of Glasgow: a weight management programme for obese patients with COVID-19 (awarded about £1 million).
- LOCOMOTION, University of Leeds: aims to establish a gold standard care pathway for long COVID syndrome, including assessment, advice, treatment and home monitoring methods (awarded £3.4 million).
- EXPLAIN (HypErpolarised Xenon Magnetic Resonance PuLmonary Imaging in PAtIeNts with long COVID), University of Oxford: to study non-hospitalised patients with breathlessness by using MRI to trace inhaled gas (awarded £1.8 million).
- CICERO project (Cognitive Impairment in long COVID: PhEnotyping and RehabilitatiOn), University College London: to study 'brain fog' (cognitive COVID) with brain imaging and to assess neuropsychological rehabilitation.

Other prominent studies on long COVID syndrome

Three important pieces of research on long COVID syndrome that focuses on hospitalised patients, children and non-hospitalised patients, respectively, include:

- PHOSP-COVID, Leicester Biomedical Research Centre: The Post-Hospitalisation COVID-19 study is a national consortium of leading researchers and clinicians across the UK working together to understand and improve long-term health outcomes in hospitalised patients with COVID-19. It aims to recruit 10,000 patients who have been hospitalised with COVID-19 illness and track them for long-term health outcomes over 18 months.
- CLoCk (Children and young people with Long COVID) study, Great Ormond Street Institute of Child Health: looks at the impact of long

COVID syndrome on mental health in children, young people and their families.

- The TLC study (Therapies for Long COVID in non-hospitalised individuals), University of Birmingham: a £2.2 million government-funded research to identify ways to improve treatment and investigate the causes and symptoms of long COVID syndrome in non-hospitalised patients.

Epidemiological studies

The NIHR and UK Research and Innovation (UKRI) have funded two research studies:

- REACT-LC (REACT-Long COVID) study, Imperial College London: data collected from more than half a million adults; over a third of those with COVID-19 reported persistent symptoms lasting more than 12 weeks, and around one in ten had severe symptoms of long COVID syndrome.
- CONVALESCENCE study, University College London and King's College London: anonymised data from 1.2 million primary care health records from across the UK, of which data on 45,096 patients were used. The incidence of long COVID syndrome was 17% in middle-aged people, falling to 7.8% in younger adults; 4.8% of middle-aged people reported long COVID syndrome affected their routine daily activities, compared to 1.2% of 20-year olds who had COVID-19, and women were 50% more likely to report long COVID symptoms than men.

Themed reviews on long COVID syndrome

The NIHR published two themed reviews by collating evidence on long COVID syndrome:

- First themed review: published in October 2020, this was the first dynamic themed review on long COVID syndrome. It highlights the need for a consensus on diagnostic criteria for persistent COVID-19 symptoms. It recognises the fluctuating and multisystemic nature of these symptoms, which, if not managed well, can lead to significant psychological and social impact and long-term consequences for individuals and society. It emphasises the need for a holistic approach, in both service provision and research.

- Second themed review: published in March 2021, this themed review focuses on published evidence from a survey of 3000 people living with long COVID syndrome. It quotes the variable estimations in the prevalence of long COVID syndrome, the growing list of symptoms associated with this condition and the fact that organ impairment occurs in both hospitalised and non-hospitalised patients. It reviews the evidence on cognitive processing disorders and anxiety, highlighting their neurological, rather than social, causes. Long COVID syndrome can be very debilitating, with 71% of respondents reporting that it affected their family life, 80% that it affected their ability to work and 36% that it affected their finances. It emphasises the need for joined-up care across specialties and between primary and secondary care, based on a multiprofessional workforce strategy. This review highlights the need for more research on long COVID syndrome, with equal partnership between researchers and patients in setting the research agenda. It also explains the need for rapid evaluation of different service models.

Research on long COVID syndrome in the United States

In February 2021, the National Institutes of Health (NIH) from the United States announced an investment of $1.15 billion in research on long COVID syndrome over 4 years. The NIH has also given details of research opportunities as part of the newly created Post-Acute Sequelae of SARS-CoV-2 infection (PASC) Initiative.

Key Points

- Research is needed on long COVID syndrome to establish evidence-based pathways for diagnosis, assessment and management of the condition.
- The UK government recognises the importance of research on long COVID syndrome and has awarded huge funding to various research groups.
- The UK has been leading the way in promoting research on long COVID syndrome since the early stages of the pandemic, realising the effects of its long-term sequelae on society.
- The NIHR has published two themed reviews on long COVID syndrome.

References

1. Department of Health and Social Care (2021). Press release: new research into treatment and diagnosis of long COVID. Available from: https://www.gov.uk/government/news/new-research-into-treatment-and-diagnosis-of-long-covid.
2. NIHR Leicester Biomedical Research Centre. PHOSP-COVID. Available from: https://www.leicesterbrc.nihr.ac.uk/themes/respiratory/research/phosp-covid/.
3. Public Health England, Great Ormond Street Institute of Child Health. Children and young people with long COVID (CLoCk). Available from: https://assets.publishing.service.gov.uk/government/uploads/system/uploads/attachment_data/file/977177/Children_and_young_people_with_Long_Covid__CLoCK_.pdf.
4. University of Birmingham. Therapies for long COVID in non-hospitalised individuals: the TLC Study. Available from: https://www.birmingham.ac.uk/research/applied-health/research/long-covid/index.aspx.
5. National Institute for Health Research (2021). Up to one in three people who have had COVID-19 report long COVID symptoms. Available from: https://www.nihr.ac.uk/news/up-to-one-in-three-people-who-have-had-covid-19-report-long-covid-symptoms/27979.
6. National Institute for Health Research (2020). Themed review: living with Covid19. Available from: https://evidence.nihr.ac.uk/themedreview/living-with-covid19/.

7.   National Institute for Health Research (2021). Themed review: living with Covid19 — second review. Available from: https://evidence.nihr.ac.uk/themedreview/living-with-covid19-second-review/.

8.   National Institutes of Health (2021). NIH launches new initiative to study 'long COVID'. Available from: https://www.nih.gov/about-nih/who-we-are/nih-director/statements/nih-launches-new-initiative-study-long-covid.

Chapter 51

New medications under investigation in trials

Introduction

There are many theoretical proposals for the efficacy of different medications in long COVID syndrome. However, these theories have to be proven by translational research in patients. Time is needed to assess whether these physio-pharmacological theories can be translated into clinically effective treatments. Although none of these new medications can be recommended for use yet, this chapter will create an awareness of the relevant trials undertaken in the context of long COVID syndrome.

CCR5 inhibitors

C-C chemokine receptor type 5 (CCR5) is a receptor via which some types of viruses enter cells, similarly to human immunodeficiency virus (HIV) infection. CCR5 blockers have been used as antivirals and have also been tried by some researchers to treat patients with long COVID syndrome, on the basis that viral particles cause persistent inflammation. However, results are awaited to show their efficacy in clinical practice.

Leronlimab is a human monoclonal antibody against CCR5 and has entered phase 2 trials at the time of writing. Studies have shown benefits of leronlimab in terms of clinical, immunological and virological parameters in acute COVID-19 illness. However, further research is needed to investigate the long-term effects of leronlimab.

Tocilizumab

Tocilizumab is a recombinant humanised monoclonal antibody that blocks the inflammatory cytokine, interleukin-6 (IL-6). It is a biological therapy used in the treatment of rheumatoid arthritis. The RECOVERY Collaborative Group trial showed that tocilizumab improved survival and clinical outcomes in hospitalised patients with acute COVID-19 who presented with hypoxia and systemic inflammation, although findings from previous trials were inconclusive.

A trial is under way investigating the role of tocilizumab in the treatment of long COVID syndrome (NCT04330638).

Colchicine

COVID-19 illness can progress in three phases:

- Early infection when the virus enters the cells.
- Pulmonary phase where the virus propagates and damages the lungs with activation of the host immune response.
- Inflammatory cascade where inflammatory mediators drive the cytokine storm despite a fall in viral titres.

Colchicine has anti-inflammatory effects and works in the third phase, causing a reduction in inflammatory mediators. Colchicine has been proposed for the treatment of pulmonary fibrosis in long COVID syndrome due to its antifibrotic effects as a microtubule-destabilising agent.

The use of colchicine has also been suggested to target neutrophil extracellular traps (NETs) in long COVID syndrome. For more details on NETs, see Chapter 45.

The RECOVERY trial found no evidence supporting the use of colchicine in hospitalised COVID-19 patients. Further phase 4 trials are planned to determine the clinical efficacy of colchicine in treating pulmonary fibrosis in patients with long COVID syndrome.

Ivermectin

Ivermectin is an antiparasitic medication used to treat river blindness. It has been proposed to treat the persistent effects of long COVID syndrome. The University of Oxford's PRINCIPLE (Platform Randomised Trial of Treatments in the Community for Epidemic and Pandemic Illnesses) trial is investigating the role of ivermectin in treating COVID-19 illness.

Recombinant DNase

Recombinant DNase is used in the treatment of cystic fibrosis. It has been suggested to have a role in reducing NETs in the sputum of patients with severe COVID-19 illness, as mass spectrometry analyses of plasma and sputum showed resolution of inflammation. Whether recombinant DNase can be used in the treatment of long COVID syndrome remains to be seen and must be based on future trials. However, it might be an expensive treatment option and needs to be trialled first.

Therapies for autoantibodies

In long COVID syndrome, studies have found that autoantibodies stimulated by COVID-19 can persist for a long time, even at 7 months post-infection. Autoantibodies are more commonly found during the recovery period in symptomatic patients, rather than in asymptomatic individuals. It has been proposed that immune modulators such as type I interferons can be useful in the treatment of long COVID syndrome.

Other experimental medications

Many medications have been trialled in research on long COVID syndrome — these include:

- Caplacizumab-yhdp is a targeted nanobody-based treatment (directed against the von Willebrand factor antibody) for thrombotic thrombocytopenic purpura (along with plasma exchange and immunosuppression); it has been used in thrombotic complications in long COVID syndrome.

- A combination of ezetimibe and atorvastatin (Atozet) is used to treat blood clotting and inflammatory disorders in long COVID syndrome.
- Ivabradine is a hyperpolarisation-activated cyclic nucleotide-gated channel blocker used to treat heart failure; it has been trialled for the treatment of postural hypotension symptoms in long COVID syndrome.
- Rintatolimod is a toll-like receptor 3 (TLR3) agonist and can reduce NET formation; it has been trialled to treat chronic fatigue.
- Montelukast is a leukotriene receptor antagonist that prevents bronchoconstriction and is used in asthma; a trial (NCT04695704) is under way to study its role in the treatment of respiratory conditions associated with long COVID syndrome.
- High-dose intravenous vitamin C is being trialled (NCT04401150) in the LOVIT-COVID study.
- Nicotinamide riboside is a dietary supplement that is currently being trialled (NCT04809974, NCT04604704) to investigate its role in treating cognitive symptoms and fatigue by modulating the pro-inflammatory response.
- Cyclic peptides that act on damage-associated molecular patterns (DAMPs) in viral infection are currently being trialled.
- Probiotic supplements are currently being trialled (NCT04813718) to determine whether the gut microbiome can be normalised and inflammation reduced in long COVID syndrome.
- Melatonin has been used in many chronic pain conditions; due to its antioxidant and anti-inflammatory effects, it could be a trial candidate for the treatment of long COVID syndrome.
- Adaptogens are derived from herbs and mushrooms, with possible health benefits in a variety of chronic conditions. It is currently being trialled (NCT04795557) as an adjuvant treatment in long COVID syndrome.
- Stem cell therapy is also in experimental use.
- Inhaled interferon therapy is being trialled in patients with lung symptoms.

- Deuterated pirfenidone has been suggested for the treatment of lung fibrosis-related symptoms.
- The drug BC007 that binds to autoantibodies against G-protein-coupled receptors (GPCRs) was originally developed for the treatment of heart failure and glaucoma; however, it has been reported to be beneficial in treating long COVID patients. A case report described improved eye symptoms, as well as full recovery from long COVID symptoms, including fatigue, loss of taste and concentration problems, within a few hours of treatment with BC007.

Key Points

- **Various new medications are being trialled for the treatment of long COVID syndrome, with some drugs tested for their anti-inflammatory effects to treat persistent inflammation and others for their antifibrotic properties to treat long COVID-associated lung fibrosis.**
- **It is too early to recommend any of these agents and proper randomised controlled trials are needed to test their efficacy.**

References

1. Patterson BK, Seethamraju H, Dhody K, *et al*. CCR5 inhibition in critical COVID-19 patients decreases inflammatory cytokines, increases CD8 T-cells, and decreases SARS-CoV2 RNA in plasma by day 14. *Int J Infect Dis* 2021; 103: 25–32.

2. Reyes AZ, Hu KA, Teperman J, *et al*. Anti-inflammatory therapy for COVID-19 infection: the case for colchicine. *Ann Rheum Dis* 2021; 80: 550–7.

3. RECOVERY Collaborative Group. Tocilizumab in patients admitted to hospital with COVID-19 (RECOVERY): a randomised, controlled, open-label, platform trial. *Lancet* 2021; 397: 1637–45.

4.   RECOVERY Collaborative Group, Horby PW, Campbell M, Spata E, *et al.* Colchicine in patients admitted to hospital with COVID-19 (RECOVERY): a randomised, controlled, open-label, platform trial. Available from: https://www.medrxiv.org/content/10.1101/2021.05.18.21257267v1.

5.   ClinicalTrials.gov. Colchicine and post-COVID-19 pulmonary fibrosis. ClinicalTrials.gov identifier: NCT04818489. Available from: https://clinicaltrials.gov/ct2/show/NCT04818489.

6.   University of Oxford. PRINCIPLE: Platform Randomised Trial of Treatments in the Community for Epidemic and Pandemic Illnesses. Available from: https://www.principletrial.org.

7.   Fisher J, Mohanty T, Karlsson CAQ, *et al.* Proteome profiling of recombinant DNase therapy in reducing NETs and aiding recovery in COVID-19 patients. *Mol Cell Proteomics* 2021; 20: 100113.

8.   Shankar K, Huffman DL, Peterson C, *et al.* A case of COVID-19 induced thrombotic thrombocytopenic purpura. *Cureus* 2021; 13: e16311.

9.   Schmidt C. COVID-19 long haulers. *Nat Biotechnol* 2021; 39: 908–13.

10. Crooke H, Raza S, Nowell J, *et al.* Long COVID — mechanisms, risk factors, and management. *BMJ* 2021; 374: n1648.

11. Friedrich-Alexander-Universität Erlangen-Nürnberg (2021). Medications for autoantibodies also effective for long COVID. Available from: https://www.fau.eu/2021/07/06/news/medication-for-autoantibodies-also-effective-for-long-covid/.

Chapter 52

Other experimental therapies

Introduction

None of the experimental therapies described in this chapter in the treatment of long COVID syndrome can be recommended as they all need to be properly researched. While some of these therapies might translate into clinical benefits, we still need to wait for trial results.

Neuromodulation therapy

The use of targeted neuromodulation technology for persistent symptoms of long COVID syndrome is currently being studied:

- Vagal nerve stimulation: transcutaneous vagal nerve stimulation (tVNS) is performed non-invasively. The technique has been studied in double-blind clinical trials. One study used a 45-minute stimulation sequence at a frequency of 25Hz and a pulse width of 250µs for 10 consecutive days, and the intensity of long COVID symptoms was scored by the patients. Results showed a positive outcome after ten sessions, with 'very significant improvement' at 1 week post-treatment. Improvements were noted in terms of fatigue as measured by the Pichot Fatigue Scale, mood as measured by the Beck Depression

Inventory, muscle strength as measured by an electronic hand dynamometer and oxygen saturation as measured by finger pulse oximetry. Another study investigated home-based transcutaneous auricular vagus nerve stimulation which has been proposed for the treatment of neuropsychiatric symptoms such as fatigue, headache and anxiety. The stimulator is wearable, with possible remote stimulation control and home-based vital sign monitoring.

- Transcranial direct current stimulation (tDCS): trials have been registered on the use of tDCS in COVID-19 whereby non-invasive brain stimulation with a low-intensity electrical current can modulate prefrontal or supplementary motor areas. These trials will study outcomes of functioning, mood, anxiety, autonomic response and motor function.
- Radioelectric asymmetric conveyer (REAC) technology: this neuromodulation technology involves two types — neuropostural optimisation (NPO) and neuropsychophysical optimisation-cervicobrachial (NPPO-CB). This technology is used to optimise environmental stressors in periods of psychosocial stress in patients with long COVID syndrome. The treatment is easy to administer and can be given to large groups of patients over a short time.

Hyperbaric oxygen

There are reports that hyperbaric oxygen has benefits in the treatment of many illnesses, although with no specific evidence. Hyperbaric oxygen is used for a number of indications (apart from its original indication of decompression sickness), including tissue healing, severe refractory infections in skin or bone, chronic ulcers, neuro-rehabilitation, migraines, chronic pain problems, etc. A trial is also under way on its use in long COVID syndrome (NCT04842448) and results are awaited.

Nanoparticle technology

Zofin is an acellular biological product that contains 300 growth factors, cytokines and chemokines derived from perinatal tissues. A phase II trial on its use for respiratory distress in COVID-19 patients is in progress. There are, however, published reports of beneficial outcomes in long-hauler patients. One case report detailed the benefits of Zofin in treating breathlessness, fatigue and muscle aches, with the long-hauler patient returning to work after 3–4 weeks.

Key Points

- Neuromodulation may have a role in treating long COVID syndrome; however, further research is needed.
- Non-invasive vagal stimulators have been tried and found to be beneficial in a small series of patients with long COVID syndrome.

References

1. Verbanck P, Clarinval AM, Burton F, et al. Transcutaneous auricular vagal nerve stimulation (tVNS) can reverse the manifestations of the long-COVID syndrome: a pilot study. Front Neurol Neurosci Res 2021; 2: 100011.

2. CISION PR Newswire (2021). Soterix medical study to address post-COVID neurological and psychiatric symptoms using at-home neuromodulation and monitoring. Available from: https://www.prnewswire.com/news-releases/soterix-medical-study-to-address-post-covid-neurological-and-psychiatric-symptoms-using-at-home-neuromodulation-and-monitoring-301215486.html.

3. ClinicalTrials.gov. Neuromodulation in COVID-19 patients. ClinicalTrials.gov identifier: NCT04808284. Available from: https://clinicaltrials.gov/ct2/show/NCT04808284.

4. Pinheiro Barcessat AR, Nolli Bittencourt M, Duarte Pereira L, et al. REAC Cervicobrachial neuromodulation treatment of depression, anxiety, and stress during the COVID-19 pandemic. Psychol Res Behav Manage 2020; 13: 929–37.

5. Crooke H, Raza S, Nowell J, et al. Long COVID — mechanisms, risk factors, and management. BMJ 2021; 374: n1648.

6.   McKenzie H (2020). Therapeutics for 'COVID-19 long-haulers' exploding onto the scene as 2020 ends. Biospace. Available from: https://www.biospace.com/article/therapeutics-for-covid-19-long-haulers-exploding-onto-the-scene-as-2020-ends/.

Index

tiredness *see* fatigue
TLC study 283
tocilizumab 62, 288
topical therapies 197, 214–15, 223
tramadol 226–7
transcranial direct current stimulation 294
transcutaneous electrical nerve stimulation (TENS) 237–9
tricyclic antidepressants 221–2, 223

UK
  economic impact 43, 44, 47
  NHS England plans and services 47, 100, 105–8, 137–41
  NICE guidelines 96–7, 111–15, 223–4, 234, 241, 242, 264–5
  prevalence 15–16, 269
  research 10, 281–4
  SIGN guidelines 125–6
  support groups 275–7
unemployment 15, 31, 45
USA
  guidelines 121–3
  research 284

vaccination 265
vagal nerve stimulation 293–4
variants of concern 5–7
vascular system 24, 59–60, 61
vitamins 189, 193, 290
vomiting 194–5

WHO (World Health Organization) 125, 127–8
women 40

yellow flags 100, 242–3
'Your COVID Recovery' online support program 143–5, 149

Zofin 294–5